# International Perspectives on Voice Disorders

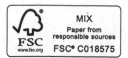

**COMMUNICATION DISORDERS ACROSS LANGUAGES**
**Series Editors:** Dr Nicole Müller and Dr Martin Ball, *University of Louisiana at Lafayette, USA*

While the majority of work in communication disorders has focused on English, there has been a growing trend in recent years for the publication of information on languages other than English. However, much of this is scattered through a large number of journals in the field of speech pathology/communication disorders, and therefore, not always readily available to the practitioner, researcher and student. It is the aim of this series to bring together into book form surveys of existing studies on specific languages, together with new materials for the language(s) in question. We also have launched a series of companion volumes dedicated to issues related to the cross-linguistic study of communication disorders. The series does not include English (as so much work is readily available), but covers a wide number of other languages (usually separately, though sometimes two or more similar languages may be grouped together where warranted by the amount of published work currently available). We have been able to publish volumes on Finnish, Spanish, Chinese and Turkish, and books on multilingual aspects of stuttering, aphasia, and speech disorders, with several others in preparation.

Full details of all the books in this series and of all our other publications can be found on http://www.multilingual-matters.com, or by writing to Multilingual Matters, St Nicholas House, 31–34 High Street, Bristol BS1 2AW, UK.

# International Perspectives on Voice Disorders

Edited by
**Edwin M-L. Yiu**

**MULTILINGUAL MATTERS**
Bristol • Buffalo • Toronto

MW

**Library of Congress Cataloging in Publication Data**
International Perspectives on Voice Disorders/Edited by Edwin M-L. Yiu.
Communication Disorders Across Languages: 9
Includes bibliographical references.
1. Voice disorders — Cross-cultural studies. I. Yiu, Edwin, 1958- editor of compilation.
RF510.I58 2013
616.85'56–dc23 2012036460

**British Library Cataloguing in Publication Data**
A catalogue entry for this book is available from the British Library.

ISBN-13: 978-1-84769-873-5 (hbk)

**Multilingual Matters**
*UK:* St Nicholas House, 31–34 High Street, Bristol BS1 2AW, UK.
*USA:* UTP, 2250 Military Road, Tonawanda, NY 14150, USA.
*Canada:* UTP, 5201 Dufferin Street, North York, Ontario M3H 5T8, Canada.

The policy of Multilingual Matters/Channel View Publications is to use papers that are
natural, renewable and recyclable products, made from wood grown in sustainable
forests. In the manufacturing process of our books, and to further support our policy,
preference is given to printers that have FSC and PEFC Chain of Custody certification.
The FSC and/or PEFC logos will appear on those books where full certification has been
granted to the printer concerned.

Typeset by Techset Composition Ltd., Salisbury, UK.
Printed and bound in Great Britain by the MPG Books Group.

6/18/13

# Contents

# Contributors

**Ofer Amir**, PhD
Department of Communication Disorders, School of Health Professions, Sackler Faculty of Medicine, Tel Aviv University, Israel
Email: oferamir@post.tau.ac.il

**Janet Baker**, PhD
Adjunct Associate Professor, Speech Pathology and Audiology, School of Medicine, Flinders University, Australia
Email: janet.baker@flinders.edu.au

**Mara Behlau**, PhD
Director, Center for Voice Studies ('Centro de Estudos da Voz' – CEV), São Paulo, Brazil
Email: mbehlau@uol.com.br

**Paul Carding**, PhD
Professor of Speech and Voice Pathology, Otolaryngology, Freeman Hospital, University of Newcastle-upon-Tyne, UK
Email: paul.carding@nuth.nhs.uk

**Marc De Bodt**, MA, PhD
Professor, University Rehabilitation Centre for Communication Disorders, Antwerp University Hospital, Belgium
Visiting Professor (Speech Pathology & Audiology), Ghent University, Ghent, Belgium
Email: Marc.de.bodt@uza.be

**Vincent Deary**
Senior Lecturer, Department of Psychology, Northumbria University, UK
Email: vincent.deary@unn.ac.uk

**Tanya L. Eadie**, PhD, CCC-SLP
Associate Professor, Department of Speech and Hearing Sciences, University
of Washington, USA
Email: teadie@u.washington.edu

**Demin Han**, MD, PhD
Professor, Department of Otorhinolaryngology – Head and Neck Surgery,
Beijing Tongren Hospital, Capital Medical University, China
Email: handm@trhos.com

**Edie R. Hapner**, PhD, CCC-SLP
Associate Professor, Otolaryngology – Head and Neck Surgery, Emory Voice
Center, Emory University, USA
Email: ehapner@emory.edu

**Shigeru Hirano**, MD, PhD
Associate Professor, Department of Otolaryngology, Faculty of Medicine,
Kyoto University, Japan
Email: hirano@ent.kuhp.kyoto-u.ac.jp

**Jiangping Kong**, PhD
Professor, Department of Chinese, Peking University, China
Email: jpkong@pku.edu.cn

**Triska K-Y. Lee**
Postgraduate Candidate, Voice Research Laboratory, Division of Speech and
Hearing Sciences, University of Hong Kong, Hong Kong
Email: triska@hku.hk

**Nicole Y-K. Li**, PhD
Visiting Assistant Scientist, Department of Surgery, University of Wisconsin-
Madison, USA
Email: nyli2@wisc.edu

**Estella P-M. Ma**, PhD
Assistant Professor, Voice Research Laboratory, Division of Speech and
Hearing Sciences, University of Hong Kong, Hong Kong
Email: estella.ma@hku.hk

**Glaucya Madazio**, PhD
Associate Professor, Center for Voice Studies ('Centro de Estudos da Voz' –
CEV), São Paulo, Brazil
Email: glaumadazio@uol.com.br

**Cate Madill**, PhD
Lecturer, Discipline of Speech Pathology, Faculty of Health Sciences, University of Sydney, Australia
Email: cate.madill@sydney.edu.au

**Youri Maryn**, MA, PhD
Professor, Department of Speech Pathology, St. Johns Hospital, Bruges, and University College Vesalius, Ghent, Belgium
Email: youri.maryn@azbrugge.be

**Patricia McCabe**, PhD
Senior Lecturer, Discipline of Speech Pathology, Faculty of Health Sciences, University of Sydney, Australia
Email: tricia.mccabe@sydney.edu.au

**Tracy Miller**
Principal Speech Therapist (Voice Disorders), Department of Otolaryngology, Freeman Hospital, UK

**Jennifer Oates**, PhD
Associate Professor, School of Human Communication Sciences, Faculty of Health Sciences, La Trobe University, Australia
Email: j.oates@latrobe.edu.au

**Gisele Oliveira**, PhD
Associate Professor, Center for Voice Studies ('Centro de Estudos da Voz' – CEV), São Paulo, Brazil
Email: giseleoliveiracev@uol.com.br

**Bernadette Timmermans**, MA, PhD
Professor, Researcher, Erasmus Hogeschool Brussels, Interdisciplinary Teacher Training Department, Free University Brussels, and Postdoctoral Researcher, Antwerp University, Belgium
Email: bernadette.timmermans@ehb.be

**Koichi Tsunoda**, MD
Department of Artificial Organs and Medical Device Creation, National Hospital Organization, National Tokyo Medical Center, National Institute of Sensory Organs, and Department of Otolaryngology, University of Tokyo, Japan
Email: tsunodakoichi@kankakuki.go.jp

**Kristiane M. Van Lierde**, MA, PhD
Professor, Researcher (Speech Pathology & Audiology), Ghent University, and Voice Clinician, Ghent University Hospital, Belgium
Email: Kristiane.vanlierde@ugent.be

**Katherine Verdolini-Abbott**, PhD, CCC-SLP
Professor, Department of Communication Science and Disorders, University of Pittsburgh, USA
Email: kav25@pitt.edu

**Anne Vertigan**, BAppSc (Sp Path), MBA, PhD
Director, Speech Pathology, Hunter New England Health, John Hunter Hospital, Australia
Email: anne.vertigan@hnehealth.nsw.gov.au

**Gaowu Wang**, PhD
Postdoctoral Fellow, Voice Research Laboratory, Division of Speech & Hearing Sciences, University of Hong Kong, Hong Kong
Email: gwwang@hku.hk

**Wen Xu**, MD, PhD
Professor, Director of Laryngology, Beijing Tongren Hospital, Capital Medical University, China
Email: xuwenlily@yahoo.com.cn

**Rosiane Yamasaki**, PhD
Associate Professor, Center for Voice Studies ('Centro de Estudos da Voz' – CEV), São Paulo, Brazil
Email: r.yamasaki@uol.com.br

**Edwin M-L. Yiu**, PhD
Professor, Voice Research Laboratory/Swallowing Research Laboratory, Division of Speech and Hearing Sciences, University of Hong Kong, Hong Kong, and Honorary Professor, Discipline of Speech Pathology, Faculty of Health Sciences, University of Sydney, Australia
Email: eyiu@hku.hk

# Preface

Best clinical practice is informed by research, and research is dependent upon the availability of resources. Clinical practice and research in voice is no exception. Large amounts of resources have been invested into voice research so that the findings and outcome can be used to inform practitioners on clinical practice.

In general, clinical practice in voice can be divided into assessment and therapy. Clinical voice assessment procedures rely on medical (anatomical and physiological) examination of the phonatory system, and subjective (auditory-perceptual) and instrumental evaluation of voice production. These assessment procedures are based on extensive experience and research findings in the acoustic, aerodynamic and physiological domains. On the other hand, voice therapy is both an art and a science, in which the therapy giver, be it a surgeon or a behavioural voice therapist, has to develop good therapeutic skills based on their scientific knowledge.

Voice research has traditionally been undertaken by large research centres or clinical facilities that are well funded financially. They are mostly found in developed countries. Nevertheless, recent developments show that voice research has been undertaken by many independent research facilities around the world and, although their funding might not be as good as those at the leading institutes, the quality of their research work is equally first class and cutting edge. It is with these in mind that a book project was formulated with the inclusion of world experts in clinical voice practice and research to contribute to a series of discussions about the best clinical practice and research in different parts of the world.

Voice experts from almost every continent – Europe, Asia, Oceania, North and South America – have contributed to this book. Part 1 covers issues of clinical practice in various countries. Both similarities and differences in clinical practice can be noted in these reports. Part 2 describes current research in the very many different countries. A number of these reports highlight some areas not undertaken by the mainstream research centres, thus demonstrating how important it is to have a contemporary understanding of a variety of research from all over the world. I would like to thank all the contributors, firstly for agreeing to contribute to this book, and secondly for writing chapters with a unified format, despite such diverse backgrounds.

EY
July 2012

# Part 1

# Current Issues in Voice Assessment and Intervention: A World Perspective

# 1 Current Issues in Voice Assessment and Intervention in Australia

## Jennifer Oates, Janet Baker and Anne Vertigan

## Introduction

Voice assessment and intervention in Australia share many features with voice practice internationally. However, because of the specific educational, public policy and cultural environment of Australia, it is likely that Australian practice is characterised by several unique features. This chapter describes the context for voice practice in Australia and discusses current practice in relation to speech pathology education, continuing professional development, service delivery and cultural influences.

Because there are limited published data on contemporary voice practice in Australia, the authors developed and implemented three surveys to ensure that the content of this chapter is as current and reflective of actual practice as possible. All three surveys were administered electronically with the target groups all being academics responsible for voice education in Australian universities, convenors of special interest groups in voice, and managers of speech pathology departments in a range of health and community agencies. The survey of academics was followed up with phone calls to explore responses in further depth.

### The context of voice practice in Australia

Australia has a population of 22.8 million people spread over 7.6 million square kilometres (just slightly smaller than the USA). Some parts of the country are very remote. Australia is a wealthy country with a GDP in 2011 of US$1.03 trillion (the 13th largest economy in the world), low unemployment (5.3%), and a 99% literacy rate (Australian Bureau of Statistics, 2012).

Mean household income is equivalent to US$61,650. Although school education is free, approximately one-third of children attend private schools. Seventy-five per cent of the population have completed 10 or more years of education and 42% of the population have completed 12 or more years. The majority of the population lives in urban areas. Health care in Australia is generally good, and life expectancy averages 81 years.

Australia has a long history of immigration with 24% of the current population having been born outside Australia. The majority of the population is monolingual and there are no recognised Australian dialects. Fifteen million Australians (68%) speak only English. Other common languages include Italian, Greek, Cantonese, Mandarin and Vietnamese. Recently, Australia has also had increased numbers of refugees from African countries, particularly Sudan. Only 2.5% of the population identify themselves as indigenous, that is Aboriginal or Torres Strait Islander. Unfortunately there is an inequitable health gap between indigenous and non-indigenous Australians and a generally low uptake of health and speech pathology services by both of these populations. Average life expectancy for indigenous Australians is approximately 70 years.

Epidemiological data on the prevalence of voice problems in Australia demonstrate that approximately 4% of the general adult population report that they experience voice problems in any one year (Russell *et al.*, 2005). The prevalence rate for occupational voice users is considerably higher than for the general population. The equivalent prevalence rate for Australian school teachers, for example, is 20% (Russell *et al.*, 1998). Few prevalence data are available for Australian children, but early parent-reported data from a large epidemiological study of 4-year-old children in Australia indicate a rate of 1.8% of 4-year-olds with a voice problem and 7% with hoarse voices (J. Skeat, personal communication, 3 August 2009).

Assessment and intervention services for people with voice problems in Australia are provided mainly by speech pathologists and otolaryngologists. Although many speech pathologists and otolaryngologists develop specialist skills in voice practice, it is rare for these health professionals to practice solely in the voice field. There are no phoniatricians in Australia and very few otolaryngologists title themselves as laryngologists. Otolaryngologists are responsible for making the medical diagnosis and for the implementation of medical and surgical intervention for people with voice disorders, but speech pathologists often assume the key coordinating role in the overall management of these clients. Speech pathologists and otolaryngologists often work closely together in client management as well as research and professional development. Other health professionals including neurologists, respiratory physicians and psychologists also contribute to the management of people with voice disorders, although not on a routine basis. In addition, singing and acting voice teachers, speaking voice coaches, physiotherapists, osteopaths and Alexander and Feldenkrais practitioners are sometimes involved in assessment and intervention.

Speech pathology in Australia is a relatively young profession, having been founded by a speech therapist from England in 1931. The first speech pathology training course commenced in 1939 as a hospital-based diploma. In 1967 the first university degree course in speech pathology commenced. As of 2010, there are 10 university degree courses that qualify graduates to practise. These qualifying or entry-level courses are offered as bachelors, bachelors/masters double degrees and graduate-entry masters degrees. It is not possible to specify the exact number of speech pathologists in Australia at the present time because speech pathology is not a nationally registered profession. However, the profession is strongly self-regulated through its professional association, Speech Pathology Australia (SPA), and eligibility for membership of SPA is normally required for employment. As of 2009, there were 4420 members. From the early days in the development of the profession in Australia, knowledge and skills in the management of people with voice disorders have been considered as key competencies for speech pathologists. SPA requires that all members are competent for voice practice and university programmes cannot be accredited by SPA unless they can demonstrate that their graduates have been assessed as being competent in voice (SPA, 2001).

# Entry-Level Preparation of Speech Pathologists for Voice Practice

Competency-based occupational standards set by SPA (2001) specify that speech pathologists who are eligible for membership of SPA must be competent to work with both adults and children in each of the five key areas of voice, speech, language, fluency and swallowing. Entry-level clinicians are expected to be competent for voice practice across seven areas of professional activity: assessment; analysis and interpretation of assessment data; intervention planning; intervention; planning, maintaining and delivering speech pathology services; professional and community education; and continuing professional development. To be accredited by SPA, university programmes must demonstrate that all graduates meet these entry-level standards.

The findings from the authors' email and telephone survey presented below provide more detailed information and qualitative insights on the education of speech pathologists than can be provided by the competency requirements outlined above. This additional information further explains the context and underpinnings of clinical practice in Australia. The survey revealed the following features of entry-level speech pathology education in voice.

## The proportion of each course devoted to voice theory

The proportion of each course devoted to voice theory ranges between 10% and 22%, with the mode being 10%. Although respondents were not asked to specify the proportions allocated to the other four areas of competency, it is clear that voice and fluency receive less attention in entry-level education than do speech, language and swallowing. Some respondents felt that the proportion of their programmes devoted to voice was too small. However, an equal number stated that the amount of their courses devoted to voice was about right because clients with voice disorders constitute a relatively small proportion of the caseloads in many clinical settings. A sense that voice problems are a lower priority than other conditions, particularly dysphagia, was also expressed by some respondents. The latter was not, however, a strong or consistent opinion from this group of academics.

## Multiple methods of learning and teaching

Several methods are employed in all the courses. That is, no one approach is the dominant method of teaching. Traditional methods such as lectures, demonstrations, tutorials, skills and laboratory classes are combined with less traditional approaches such as problem-based and case-based learning, workshops, online teaching and simulation approaches. The most common methods used are lectures, demonstrations and case-based learning.

## A range of diagnostic classifications for voice disorders

Diagnostic classifications for voice disorders are taught with all courses, drawing on multiple approaches to classification (most commonly, Aronson & Bless, 2009; Baker et al., 2007; Boone et al., 2005; Colton et al., 2006; Mathieson, 2001; Rammage et al., 2001; Verdolini et al., 2005). Most do not require that students use a particular published system.

## Auditory-perceptual voice analysis system

The primary auditory-perceptual voice analysis system taught in all Australian courses is the Perceptual Voice Profile (Oates & Russell, 1998). However, students in all courses are also exposed to a range of other systems including CAPE-V (Kempster et al., 2009), GRBAS (Hirano, 1981), Stockholm Voice Evaluation Approach (Hammarberg & Gauffin, 1995), and the Buffalo III Voice Profile (Wilson, 1987). Students' perceptual evaluation skills are formally assessed in most courses, normally via a listening test on standard voice samples.

## Instrumentation for voice evaluation

A range of instrumentation for voice evaluation is used in all courses. Students are exposed to instrumentation though either hands-on practice or via demonstration. Exposure is greatest for commercially available acoustic analysis systems such as the KayPENTAX tools (e.g. Computerised Speech Laboratory), downloadable acoustic analysis programs such as PRAAT, and laryngeal endoscopy and stroboscopy. Few courses provide experience with high-speed vocal fold imaging, electroglottography or aerodynamic analysis systems. The amount of exposure to instrumentation varies considerably, with a range of 1–7 hours. Although several academics stated that they had a good range of voice analysis tools, others expressed the desire to acquire further instrumentation, for increased technical support and for their students to be given greater access to instrumentation for practice in their own time. For a small number of respondents, the wish for greater access to instrumentation was tempered by the comment that by no means all clinicians in the field have access to instrumentation, the implication being that perhaps extensive training on instrumentation is not warranted in entry-level courses.

## Wide range of voice therapy techniques

Various voice therapy techniques are covered in theory classes and demonstrations in all courses. Virtually every voice therapy technique documented in the literature is covered, including programmatic methods such as Lee Silverman Voice Therapy, Lessac–Madsen Resonant Voice Therapy and Vocal Function Exercises, holistic approaches such as the Accent Method, as well as the more recently promoted vocal tract semi-occlusion exercises. Specific hands-on training is provided, but for a limited number of techniques (mostly respiratory control exercises, head and neck relaxation, resonance methods and vocal endurance/flexibility techniques). While students in several courses are required to demonstrate basic competence in using one or two voice therapy techniques through a viva voce, this is not the case for every course and few courses require students to demonstrate competence in using more than one or two therapy methods. Several academics commented that intervention skills are mostly evaluated during clinical placements rather than during the theory course and that there is little time available in the theory course to assess students' competence in voice therapy.

## Clinical experience in voice

Clinical experience in voice practice is provided for most students in all courses, either in a specialist voice clinic (for up to 40% of students) or via general placements where clients present with voice problems in conjunction with their primary speech, language or swallowing problems (for 60–100% of students). For students who do not gain voice experience in their clinical placements, a standardised patient, video or simulated patient programme is implemented. Voice experience is gained mainly in health settings and university clinics with patients having a wide range of functional and organic voice disorders. Although paediatric clinical experience in voice is provided in several courses, adult experience is far more common.

## Health promotion/prevention in the voice area

Prevention is important, therefore health promotion/prevention in the voice area is addressed in all courses. While not all programmes provide opportunities for every student to participate in health promotion/prevention activities, most students have the option to undertake a health promotion project as part of their theory course. They may also participate in health promotion activities while undertaking clinical placements, or observe an experienced clinician deliver voice care education and training to occupational voice users.

## Opportunity for students to undertake training of their own voices

This type of experience is not common, but most respondents stated that they would like to provide students with such training. Three university programmes require all students to undergo a small amount (2–4 hours) of group training of their own voices. The main reason cited for not providing voice training to students was the lack of time in the curriculum. Most academics reported, however, that they notify students of any voice training workshops offered in the community and that they encourage students to participate.

## Speech pathologists with substantial clinical and/or voice research expertise

Experienced speech pathologists are invited to teach the voice components of entry-level speech pathology courses in all universities. While half of the Australian university programmes have a voice expert on the staff, the remainder employ their voice teaching staff on a casual basis. The universities employing casual teaching staff do so because they have found it difficult to attract experienced individuals to substantive academic roles and/or because the programme has a relatively small student load that makes employing an academic with voice experience on a permanent basis less viable.

## Research and evidence-based practice in voice

Research and evidence-based practice in voice are integrated and emphasised within all programmes. Several programmes also devote teaching time to evidence-based practice issues in voice through separate research-based subjects. In this case, the focus is usually on evidence for the effectiveness of voice therapy methods. The academics' responses on their own opportunities to undertake research in the voice field were, however, more variable. Several academics reported that their positions provide considerable scope for them to undertake research; these academics were those employed in substantive positions. Those employed on a casual basis reported that there is limited opportunity for them to conduct research, although some do assist in the supervision of research students and one individual is able to undertake research outside her university role (through a government-funded centre for clinical research excellence).

In general, the academics responsible for voice education in Australian universities reported that their voice programmes are of high quality and that graduates have the strong theoretical understanding required for practice. They felt that the main factors contributing to the quality of education in voice are the extensive and current clinical experience of teaching staff, the explicit links made between theory and practice, the availability of good quality clinical case examples on DVD/video, and the high quality of the training provided in auditory-perceptual evaluation of voice. However, all of these academics stated that they would like to be able to provide increased opportunities for hands-on practice of voice therapy techniques and more clinical placements in voice for their students.

## Post-Entry Level Practice

Specialisation in voice is not common among newly graduated speech pathologists in Australia. Instead, new graduates are encouraged to seek employment across a range of public sector settings including acute hospitals, rehabilitation centres, education departments, community and mental health services, and centres for children with hearing impairment and other disabilities. Although a substantial number of new graduates are interested in undertaking specialist voice practice, most do not commence such practice until they have several years of more general experience.

Specialist multidisciplinary voice clinics have been established in a number of major teaching hospitals throughout Australia (e.g. in Adelaide, Brisbane, Melbourne and Sydney). The primary focus of these clinics tends to be on the assessment and diagnosis of voice disorders rather than on the provision of outpatient services for treatment. It may be that this limitation on the provision of outpatient voice services underlies the tradition in Australia for speech pathologists with a special interest in voice to work in private practice.

## Post-Entry Level Education

Professional development activities have been integral to furthering the specialty of voice in Australia, some of which have been achieved through the Australian Voice Association (AVA) and local Voice Interest Groups.

Voice Interest Groups provide regular opportunities to promote case discussions, workshops, seminars and master classes by national and international voice specialists. While the authors' survey of these groups has shown that these activities are avidly sought after and strongly supported in some parts of the country, in others, the Voice Interest Groups report difficulties in sustaining their membership and momentum. Anecdotal comments from colleagues around the world suggest that this may be an inevitable consequence of the alternative professional development opportunities now being provided by the many international voice symposia around the world.

Originally inspired by the Voice Foundation in the USA, the multidisciplinary AVA was established in 1991 with the aims of promoting the voice field in Australia, facilitating collaboration among all voice disciplines, promoting education and training in voice care, vocal performance and voice science, and facilitating voice research. Australian Voice Symposia organised by the AVA over the last 20 years have been primary sources for professional development for Australian voice practitioners.

Australian and international scientific meetings have provided a pivotal forum for Australian voice specialists to present their research and to attend workshops and seminars run by leaders in the field. Encouraged by the burgeoning knowledge and diversity of expertise, most Australian clinicians and vocal pedagogues specialising in voice regularly attend these conferences. Many in Australia have also undertaken further training in the use and development of their own voices with singing and acting teachers, some have undertaken international travelling fellowships, some have sought advanced-level training and qualifications in counselling and psychotherapy, while others have undertaken research and higher degrees leading to masters, doctoral and post-doctoral qualifications. There is now substantial expertise among voice specialists and, considering the relatively small size of the voice profession in Australia, there is a relatively good research output.

## Voice research in Australia

Australian speech pathologists have made a strong contribution to the voice literature with high-quality research conducted across a wide range of areas. For example, Australian studies have been reported in the international literature in the areas of neurophysiology (Davis et al., 1996), respiratory-phonatory coordination (Winkworth et al., 1994), auditory-perceptual evaluation (Oates & Russell, 1998), instrumental assessment (Madill et al., 2010; Pemberton et al., 1993; Vogel & Morgan, 2009) and diagnostic classification systems (Baker et al., 2007). There has been a strong research focus on voice disorders associated with neurological conditions (Theodoros & Murdoch, 1994; Sheard et al., 1991) and recent studies on occupational voice disorders have focused on both prevalence (Phyland et al., 1999; Russell et al., 2005) and prevention (Pasa et al., 2007). Studies have also been published in the areas of chronic cough (Vertigan et al., 2006), paradoxical vocal fold movement (Vertigan et al., 2007), transsexual voice (Carew et al., 2007), telemedicine approaches to vocal rehabilitation (Theodoros et al., 2006) and psychogenic voice disorders

(Baker, 2008, 2010; Baker & Lane, 2009). In conjunction with voice scientists and performing arts companies, speech pathologists in Australia also have reported research on acoustic features of singing and acting voice (Barnes *et al.*, 2004; Pinczower & Oates, 2005; Reid *et al.*, 2007; Walzak *et al.*, 2008).

## Future directions in post-entry level voice education

The authors' survey of voice academics, Voice Interest Groups and department managers suggests that, if increased numbers of clinicians are to progress beyond entry-level competency in the voice field, it will be necessary to encourage recently qualified practitioners to undertake further professional development, to become more actively involved in research, and to promote the general profile of voice in the profession and community. There are a small number of Australian voice practitioners in speech pathology with postgraduate research qualifications at masters and doctoral levels. Postgraduate coursework studies that would allow progression from postgraduate certificates and/or diplomas through to clinical and/or professional doctorates would also provide education leading to advanced-level practice in research literacy, clinical assessment and intervention. It is suggested that such advanced-level education and training could include more detailed attention to areas such as: instrumentation for voice assessment and therapy; competency training for laryngeal endoscopy and stroboscopy; evidence-based practice in voice; psychological interviewing and intervention; medico-legal aspects of voice practice; and complex and challenging voice disorders.

# The Australian Health System

Australia has a two-tiered health system: public and private. Public health services are provided to all Australians regardless of income or private health insurance status. Primary medical services are funded by Medicare which is partly funded by a 1.5% income tax levy. The government pays a large percentage of the cost of services in public hospitals, and 75–85% of outpatient and specialist services. The patient must pay the remainder of the service (co-payment) unless they are classified as a low-income earner. Patients may elect to take out private health insurance or pay for private services.

# Voice Services in Australia

## Medical services

In order to understand service provision in the area of voice in Australia it is necessary to understand the structures in which medical practitioners and speech pathologists are employed. The majority of medical practitioners are either Primary Care Physicians (e.g. general practitioners), or Medical Specialists. Medical Specialists may be employed in either public hospitals or private practice. Some Medical Specialists in private practice also have consulting rights to public hospitals. In addition, Primary Care Physicians may be responsible for inpatient care in small rural hospitals.

There may be limited access to medical services including otolaryngologists, particularly in rural areas. Otolaryngologists are primarily located in major capital cities or large regional centres. Patients in rural and remote areas may have to travel for several hours to access otolaryngology services. Therefore, most voice patients are seen in generalist otolaryngology outpatient clinics rather than specialist voice clinics. In fact some may only receive mirror laryngoscopy. It should also be noted that only a small number of otolaryngologists in Australia conduct phonosurgery.

## Speech pathology services

Speech pathology services can be accessed through either public or private systems. Public services are available free of charge to the vast majority of the population regardless of health insurance status, although the breadth of assessment and extent of therapy may be limited and there may be long waiting times. Private health insurance rebates reimburse a proportion of the costs for private voice services and also have an annual capping limit. Therefore patients incur a significant proportion of the cost of therapy. Patients can elect to fund the full cost of treatment after the annual capping limit has been reached. There are a number of highly specialised voice clinicians in each state in Australia. Despite this, there is a limited critical mass of speech pathologists with voice expertise.

Speech pathologists are rarely employed in private otolaryngology practices. More commonly, patients are assessed by an otolaryngologist and then referred to a speech pathologist in a different service. Strong working relationships are often developed, yet there are instances where there is limited understanding of the role and skill base of the speech pathologist and limited capacity for multidisciplinary collaboration about patient care. This can lead to a low referral rate of voice patients in some areas.

Many speech pathology services in the public and private sectors can be accessed without medical referral. There can be pressure placed on therapists to provide assessment prior to otolaryngology examination, particularly if there is difficulty in accessing otolaryngology services.

Laryngeal endoscopy is primarily the domain of otolaryngologists in Australia, despite the fact that endoscopy is considered by SPA to be within the scope of practice. There is difficulty in obtaining endoscopy for biofeedback and in-depth timely analysis of phonatory function. This lack of availability makes it difficult to diagnose and treat some disorders.

## Specialist voice clinics

High-quality voice services are readily available in metropolitan areas and in some regional areas. Australia boasts some centres of excellence in the area of multidisciplinary voice practice. These specialist clinics are staffed by speech pathologists and otolaryngologists. In some instances these clinics also engage neurologists, psychologists and singing pedagogues. Joint assessment including laryngeal endoscopy is conducted and the clinicians also collaborate on management planning. Videostroboscopy is not available outside capital city areas. Following assessment in a specialist voice clinic, clients may be referred to their local area for continued treatment by a generalist speech pathologist.

## Voice services in generalist speech pathology clinics

A substantial proportion of voice services are provided by generalist clinicians. Due to the large geographical distances and the small population, many speech pathologists are employed in sole generalist positions. They are responsible for patients within a particular geographical area across the age spectrum regardless of diagnosis. They are expected to develop wide ranging, general skills across all areas of practice. Therefore the quality of service provided may be dependent upon the individual speech pathologist's previous education, training, experience and the networks used for professional support. There is generally a good network for specialist support in the area of voice. However, despite being required to provide voice services, clinicians can experience difficulty in accessing funding and time for professional development.

Instrumental voice equipment is rarely available in generalist clinics. Fortunately, there is an emphasis on auditory perceptual voice analysis in Australia, and speech pathologists typically have strong skills in this key type of analysis. Australia developed, for example, the Perceptual Voice Profile as detailed in the CD-ROM training package *A Sound Judgement* (Oates & Russell, 1998).

## Voice services in rural areas

There is a discrepancy in the availability of voice services between metropolitan and rural areas. It is often difficult to recruit speech pathologists in rural areas, particularly those with specific experience in voice practice. Further, otolaryngologists are rarely based in rural areas and those who provide services in such areas on a visiting basis are not generally specialists in voice. Although small rural areas may never have the resources to offer specialist voice clinics, they are often able to manage voice clients well in generalist clinics with support from nearby specialist centres. However, distance and travel costs sometimes impede access to these specialist clinics for assessment.

The advent of telemedicine in speech pathology and voice practice more generally has significant ramifications for the delivery of voice services in rural areas in the future. It is already used extensively in some centres and is attracting government funding. It has the potential to increase access to voice services and to facilitate ongoing therapy and second opinions (Theodoros, 2008).

## Voice services in the public health sector

The provision of voice services in the public sector is variable. There is no national consensus about the most appropriate setting for voice services in public health, nor the prerequisite skills required to provide such a service. Voice services can be accessed in the majority of settings, but the scope and timeliness of access is limited. For example, patients may be seen for diagnosis and assessment but have difficulty in accessing ongoing therapy in their local area. In addition, some clinicians feel they are not skilled enough to deal with voice caseloads so will often refer to a specialist voice clinic.

Paediatric voice services differ between Australian states and between centres in each state. The majority of paediatric voice services are provided by generalist clinicians who work across the spectrum of early intervention, school-aged speech, language and learning disabilities, stuttering and feeding. There are a limited number of speech pathologists who specialise in paediatric voice. In some states all paediatric services are provided by Health agencies while others are provided by the Department of Education. The latter services have more emphasis on language, speech and learning disabilities and the impact of speech and language disorders in the classroom. There are a small number of specialist multidisciplinary voice services in children's hospitals in major cities. However, the majority of children are seen by speech pathologists who do not specialise in voice.

## Prioritisation of voice services in the public health sector

The extent to which voice services are prioritised in the public sector varies considerably between agencies. Each agency individually determines the relative priority of voice services. As expected, centres with specialist voice clinics tend to prioritise voice services, but some of those without such clinics also provide an accessible and substantial voice service. In general, the relative priority given to voice services depends on the patient's vocational needs, the severity of their condition and its impact on the individual's functioning.

Limitations on the types of voice problems that can be managed are sometimes imposed by the public health system. Some agencies assign voice disorders low priority if they do not meet strict referral or funding criteria, are not related to a medical condition or do not require multidisciplinary rehabilitation. Outpatient waiting lists fluctuate depending on the number of speech pathology staff vacancies. In times of staff shortage, it is often voice services that are sacrificed. Some of these limitations may also be imposed by speech pathologists themselves as they attempt to prioritise diverse and very large caseloads. Voice problems may then receive low priority in comparison to dysphagia in the acute hospital setting or to speech and language intervention in community health centres.

Despite the high demand for voice services, voice disorders are not considered a significant clinical issue in some agencies. This means that some hospitals allocate only limited speech pathology hours for voice services. In fact, health service management occasionally gives no priority at all to voice patients. Further, in one state, there is a proposal to move voice services from hospitals into the community health sector where voice assessment and intervention would be provided by generalist clinicians. Longer waiting times would be highly likely should this proposal be widely implemented.

Many speech pathologists believe, however, that voice services should be considered core business within the public health system due to the negative impact of voice disorders on quality of life and their potential to exacerbate other health and social problems. This view proposes that voice services should be available across the spectrum of prevention, early intervention and therapy. They also consider that specialist voice clinics should be available publicly in all major health agencies, particularly those with a specialist otolaryngology service, and that voice management should be part of the speech pathology management of inpatients. The impact of voice disorders on individuals, however, is not necessarily appreciated by funders, so voice services are not currently a high priority in the Australian public health system.

## Cultural Factors Impacting on Voice Practice in Australia

### Immigration patterns

Recent census data show that the pattern of migration to Australia has changed over the last 10 years (Australian Government, Department of Immigration and Citizenship, 2012). While 10% of immigrants are from the UK and Ireland, there has been a substantial decrease in migrants from Europe (from 12% down to 5%) with an increase in the 'skill stream' from Southern and Central Asia (from 7% up to 14%). However, although it is acknowledged that Australia is a multicultural society and that the migration pattern has recently changed, there is surprisingly little evidence on the impact this may be having on the prevalence and/or clinical picture of individuals presenting with voice disorders.

One of the most significant changes has been the increase in migrants seeking refugee status in Australia from countries such as Eastern Europe, the Sudan and Iraq following significant famine, political unrest and civil war, even genocide and torture. It is recognised by the Australian Department of Immigration that such traumatic and stressful circumstances can have direct effects on general physical and mental health, but to the best of the authors' knowledge, there has been no systematic investigation as to whether migrants seeking political asylum and refugee status present with voice disorders in higher numbers relative to the general population of Australia. One possible explanation for this may be that loss of voice or changes in vocal quality may not be construed as a significant health condition when considered in comparison to the basic requirements for food, water and shelter, employment and emotional support.

However, recent anecdotal data from paediatric clinicians conducting screening programmes for communication disorders in pre-school children in South Australia have revealed an interesting trend. Clinical observation suggests that a high proportion of children from families seeking asylum attending inner-city pre-school centres present not only with severe speech and language disorders, but also with significant voice disorders characterised by marked voice quality impairment. Children from countries with extremes of poverty such as Sudan, or intractable political unrest such as Iraq are commonly being identified as having what appear to be functional voice disorders. While such observations can only be regarded as anecdotal evidence, this would be a fruitful area for further research – not only among migrants seeking refugee status in Australia, but also among those searching for secure residence in other countries in the world.

## Cultural factors

There is little formal evidence to support the need for different approaches to speech pathology intervention according to the many cultural differences that characterise the Australian population (e.g. different countries of origin, religious beliefs, cultural practices and languages). At a most basic level, it is appreciated that different values in relation to gender need to be taken into account when female clinicians work with male clients from other cultures. It is understood that there are different values and boundaries assumed between females and males regardless of professional status, and that, whereas physical contact with clients in the context of carrying out voice therapy may be considered 'normal' for Australian clinicians with Australian-born clients, this may be considered totally inappropriate when working with clients from the Middle East or other Asian cultures. Investigation of the influence of cultural factors on the management of people with voice disorders is likely to be a fruitful area for future research.

## References

Aronson, A.E. and Bless, D.M. (2009) *Clinical Voice Disorders* (4th edn). New York: Thieme.
Australian Bureau of Statistics (2012) Online document, accessed 13 March 2012. http://www.abs.gov.au/AUSSTATS/abs@.nsf/mf/1345.0

Australian Government, Department of Immigration and Citizenship (2012) Online document, accessed 13 March 2012. http://www.immi.gov.au/media/statistics/country-profiles/

Baker, J. (2008) The role of psychogenic and psychosocial factors in the development of functional voice disorders. *International Journal of Speech-Language Pathology* 10, 210–230.

Baker, J. (2010) Women's voices: Lost or mislaid, stolen or strayed? *International Journal of Speech-Language Pathology* 12, 94–106.

Baker, J. and Lane, R.D. (2009) Emotion processing deficits in functional voice disorders. In K. Izdebski (ed.) *Emotions in the Human Voice, Vol. 3: Culture and Perception* (pp. 105–136). San Diego: Plural Publishing.

Baker, J., Ben-Tovim, D.I., Butcher, A., Esterman, A. and McLaughlin, K. (2007) Development of a modified diagnostic classification system for voice disorders with inter-rater reliability study. *Logopedics Phoniatrics Vocology* 32, 99–112.

Barnes, J., Davis, P., Oates, J. and Chapman, J. (2004) The relationship between professional operatic soprano voice and high range spectral energy. *Journal of the Acoustical Society of America* 116, 530–538.

Boone, D.R., McFarlane, S.C. and Von Berg, S.L. (2005) *The Voice and Voice Therapy* (7th edn). Boston, MA: Allyn & Bacon.

Carew, L., Dacakis, G. and Oates, J. (2007) The effectiveness of oral resonance therapy on the perception of femininity of voice in male-to-female transsexuals. *Journal of Voice* 21, 591–603.

Colton, R.H., Casper, J.K. and Leonard, R. (2006) *Understanding Voice Problems. A Physiological Perspective for Diagnosis and Treatment* (3rd edn). Philadelphia: Lippincott Williams and Wilkins.

Davis, P.J., Zhang, S.P., Winkworth, A. and Bandler, R. (1996) Neural control of vocalisation: Respiratory and emotional influences. *Journal of Voice* 10, 23–38.

Hammarberg, B. and Gauffin, J. (1995) Perceptual and acoustic characteristics of quality differences in pathological voices as related to physiological aspects. In O. Fujimura and M. Hirano (eds) *Vocal Fold Physiology: Voice Quality Control* (pp. 283–303). San Diego: Singular.

Hirano, M. (1981) *Clinical Examination of Voice*. New York: Springer-Verlag.

Kempster, G.B., Gerratt, B.R., Verdolini Abbott, K., Barkmeier-Kraemer, J. and Hillman, R.E. (2009) Consensus auditory-perceptual evaluation of voice: Development of a standardized clinical protocol. *American Journal of Speech-Language Pathology* 18, 124–132.

Madill, C., Sheard, C. and Heard, R. (2010) Differentiated vocal tract control and the reliability of interpretations of nasendoscopic assessment. *Journal of Voice* 24, 337–345.

Mathieson, L. (2001) *Greene and Mathieson's The Voice and Its Disorders* (6th edn). London: Whurr Publishers.

Oates, J.M. and Russell, A. (1998) Learning voice analysis using an interactive multimedia package: Development and preliminary evaluation. *Journal of Voice* 12, 500–512.

Pasa, G., Oates, J. and Dacakis, G. (2007) The relative effectiveness of vocal hygiene training and vocal function exercises in preventing voice disorders in primary school teachers. *Logopedics Phoniatrics Vocology* 32, 128–140.

Pemberton, C., Russell, A., Priestley, J., Havas, T., Hooper, J. and Clark, P. (1993) Characteristics of normal larynges under flexible fiberscopic and stroboscopic examination: An Australian perspective. *Journal of Voice* 7, 382–389.

Phyland, D.J., Oates, J.M. and Greenwood, K.M. (1999) Self-reported voice problems among three groups of professional singers. *Journal of Voice* 13, 602–611.

Pinczower, R. and Oates, J. (2005) Vocal projection in actors: The long-term average spectral features that distinguish comfortable acting voice from voicing with maximal projection in male actors. *Journal of Voice* 19, 440–453.

Rammage, L., Morrison, M. and Nichol, H. (2001) *Management of the Voice and its Disorders* (2nd edn). San Diego: Singular.

Reid, K., Davis, P., Oates, J., Cabrera, D., Ternström, S., Black, M., *et al.* (2007) The acoustic characteristics of professional opera singers performing in chorus versus solo mode. *Journal of Voice* 21, 35–45.

Russell, A., Oates, J.M. and Greenwood, K. (1998) Prevalence of voice problems in school teachers. *Journal of Voice* 12, 467–479.

Russell, A., Oates, J. and Greenwood. K. (2005) Prevalence of self-reported voice problems in the general population in South Australia. *International Journal of Speech-Language Pathology* 7, 24–30.

Sheard, C., Adams, R.D. and Davis, P.J. (1991) Reliability and agreement of ratings of ataxic dysarthric speech samples with varying intelligibility. *Journal of Speech and Hearing Research* 34, 285–293.

SPA (Speech Pathology Australia) (2001) *Competency-Based Occupational Standards (CBOS) for Speech Pathologists*. Melbourne: Author.

Theodoros, D.G. (2008) Telerehabilitation for service delivery in speech-language pathology. *Journal of Telemedicine and Telecare* 14, 221–224.

Theodoros, D.G. and Murdoch, B.E. (1994) Laryngeal dysfunction in dysarthric speakers following severe closed-head injury. *Brain Injury* 8, 667–684.

Theodoros, D.G., Constantinescu, G., Russell, T.G., Ward, E.C., Wilson, S.J. and Wootton, R. (2006) Treating the speech disorder in Parkinson's disease online. *Journal of Telemedicine and Telecare* 12 (Suppl. 3), 88–91.

Verdolini, K., Rosen, C.A. and Branski, R.C. (2005) Classification manual for voice disorders – I. Mahwah: Lawrence Erlbaum Associates.

Vertigan, A.E., Theodoros, D.G., Gibson, P.G. and Winkworth, A.L. (2006) Efficacy of speech pathology management for chronic cough: A randomized placebo controlled trial of treatment efficacy. *Thorax* 61, 1065–1069.

Vertigan, A.E., Theodoros, D.G., Gibson, P.G. and Winkworth, A. (2007) Voice and upper airway symptoms in people with chronic cough and paradoxical vocal fold movement. *Journal of Voice* 21, 361–383.

Vogel, A.P. and Morgan, A.T. (2009) Factors affecting the quality of sound recording for speech and voice analysis. *International Journal of Speech-Language Pathology* 11, 431–437.

Walzak, P., McCabe, P., Madill, C. and Sheard, C. (2008) Acoustic changes in student actors' voices after 12 months of training. *Journal of Voice* 22, 300–313.

Wilson, D.K. (1987) *Voice Problems of Children* (3rd edn). Baltimore: Williams and Wilkins.

Winkworth, A.L., Davis, P.J., Ellis, E. and Adams, R.D. (1994) Variability and consistency in speech breathing during reading: Lung volumes, speech intensity, and linguistic factors. *Journal of Speech and Hearing Research* 37, 535–556.

# 2 Current Issues in Voice Assessment and Intervention in Belgium

## Marc S. De Bodt, Bernadette Timmermans and Kristiane M. Van Lierde

Voice research in Belgium is almost completely limited to the last two decades and focused initially on the development of a widely accepted assessment protocol and the collection of reliable reference data for voice (acoustic and aerodynamic) measurements for different groups of voice users (Decoster & Debruyne, 1997a, 1997b; Morsomme, 2001; van de Heyning *et al.*, 1996).

After the turn of the century, the issue of the effectiveness of voice training and voice therapy attracted more interest, and a considerable amount of research has been done. This chapter reviews a number of projects that were realised. This provides more insight on the impact of (1) voice training and vocal warm-up programmes; (2) preventive strategies; and (3) voice therapy on the voice and voice disorders in contemporary clinical practices.

## Voice Therapy, Voice Training and the Prevention of Voice Problems in Belgium

The goal, the timing and the setting of voice therapy, voice training and the prevention of voice problems are completely different (see Table 2.1). Voice therapy is intended for dysphonic patients, is individually organised and completely voluntary. The aim is to treat the disorder and it focuses on a long-term effect. In Belgium, voice therapy tends to last for a relatively long period due to excellent reimbursement facilities. Voice training, on the other hand, is set up to improve the functioning of the (non-pathological) voice. The result of the training should be an improved voice quality and better protection against subsequent voice problems. This focus is also long-term.

**Table 2. 1** Goal, timing and setting of voice therapy, voice training and prevention of voice problems

|  | *Voice therapy* | *Voice training* | *Prevention of voice problems* |
|---|---|---|---|
| Goal 1 | Healing of the current voice disorder | Improvement of vocal functioning | Prevention of future voice problem/ disorder |
| Goal 2 | Improvement of vocal functioning/quality | Prevention of future voice problems | |
| Goal 3 | Aims for long-term effect | Aims for long-term effect | Aims for long-term effect |
| Population | Patients with voice disorders | Students with future artistic profession | Students with future voice-demanding profession |
| Timing | Very time consuming | Time restricted: 30 hours indirect and 30 hours direct | Very short: 3 hours indirect and 3 hours indirect |
| Setting | Individual approach | Very small groups (five to eight students) | Combination of small (20 students) and large groups |
| Status | Not mandatory | Mandatory | Mandatory |

Voice training is mostly organised in small groups and is limited in time. As the aim is to focus on a long-term effect, voice training is mostly spread over three years. Up to the present time there has been a tradition of voice training being part of artistic education. Since it is included in the training programme, it is therefore mandatory.

Prevention programmes, on the other hand, are primarily set up to prevent future voice problems. If the functioning of the voice also improves, this will be considered an added bonus. At present, prevention programmes are very rare and are occasionally set up in teacher training programmes. As the number of students is mostly large, it is necessary to organise the sessions for large groups (e.g. indirect training: 100 students; direct training: 20 students). Prevention programmes are mandatory for these students, limited to a few hours and mostly restricted to master's degree programmes. To our knowledge, no research has been reported about the long-term effects of prevention programmes. At present, the question of whether voice training and prevention programmes really reduce the risks for subsequent voice problems during a professional career remains unanswered. It is also unclear as to what extent the results are influenced by the obligatory nature of the programmes. It may be expected that well-motivated subjects (like patients), asking for help, show a higher interest and compliance.

On the other hand, a number of authors have demonstrated the short-term impact of voice training and vocal hygiene on the vocal performance of future vocal professionals (Berlinger & Bergin, 2005; Bovo et al., 2007; Chan, 1994; Kaufman & Johnson, 1991; Pasa et al., 2007; Roy et al., 2004; Schneider & Bigenzahn, 2005; Simberg, 2004).

# Effectiveness of Voice Training

Timmermans et al. (2004a) investigated the effectiveness of 18 months of voice training in a trained group (86 actors and radio directors) and an untrained group (103 TV and film directors). Every student was assessed by means of the multidimensional European Laryngological Society (ELS) test battery (Dejonckere et al., 2001) and a questionnaire on daily habits. More details of this study can be found in the papers by Timmermans et al. (2002, 2003b, 2004a, 2004b).

The voice training protocol consisted of theoretical lectures on 'Voice and Technique' (indirect training) in the first year. The lectures amounted to 30 hours over a period of 9 months. Following this, technical workshops (direct training) were organised. Students were trained in the use of their voices in groups of five to eight individuals. The parameters of the voice training were presented in a strict order. The second school year again included technical workshops amounting to 30 hours and students were evaluated by means of performance tasks.

The results after 9 and 18 months of voice training were clearly positive. The voice quality – calculated by means of the Dysphonic Severity Index (DSI; Wuyts et al., 2000) improved significantly from 2.3 to 4.6. This amelioration was caused by training (interaction effect was significant at $p = 0.014$). The DSI of the untrained group improved slightly from 3 to 3.7. In spite of the improved DSI score of the trained group, the perceptual evaluation remained practically identical. This is probably due to scale effects, as the G score (overall grade of hoarseness; Hirano, 1990) is not designed to score minimal changes in voice quality. The Voice Handicap Index (VHI) scores (De Bodt et al., 2000) improved in both groups but remained high, with higher scores meaning more handicapped (trained group from 18 to 14; untrained group from 20 to 15). The improvement was significant in the trained group only and was not caused by training but influenced by time only. These VHI scores show that students experience their own voices as a problem even after 18 months of voice training.

The results of this study were compared with the results of a control group, 68 pathology-free subjects with a $G_0$-score (Van de Heyning et al., 1996). The conclusion was that the voices of the future professional voice users were not as good as expected. The average DSI score of the trained group was 2, whereas the average DSI score of the control group was 5.

At the beginning of the study, videolaryngostroboscopy detected that 21% of the trained subjects were suffering from organic lesions and 27% from inflammatory lesions (oedema, erythema). The perceptual evaluation ranged from $G_0$ to $G_2$, a confirmation of the DSI score and the detected voice problems. The VHI scores supported these conclusions and indicated that the students experienced their voices as problematic. The results of the questionnaire on daily habits confirmed this negative tendency again. Smoking prevalence was high (62%); 20% of the students admitted vocal abuse and 21% of them reported that they often ate late due to scholarly or cultural activities. The voice of the future voice professional was not in good shape.

The results of this study suggested that these students did not choose the acting profession just because of their 'excellent' voice qualities. It is true that nowadays the acting population is not searching for beauty and perfection. Aesthetic criteria differ among populations of vocal professionals. Actors need to concentrate on a performance where a vivid imagination is the priority. Radio directors and radio presenters need beautiful and warm voices. Radio voices need charisma, where a slightly nasal and muffled voice is experienced as very pleasant. In other words, the criteria for an artistic-sounding voice are different from that for a healthy voice where we expect a good voice quality.

This study shows that voice training is effective, even with a rather restricted content. Further research is necessary to improve the vocal hygiene approach that has been shown to be not very effective in this study.

## Prevention Programmes

Few prevention programmes are designed for teachers and future teachers. The literature reveals some studies in which a rather short voice training programme for future teachers resulted in objectively obtained voice improvements (Duffy & Hazlett, 2004; Schneider & Bigenzahn, 2005; Simberg, 2004).

The study by Timmermans et al. (2011) investigated a cost-effective voice training module for students on an academic teacher training programme. Subjects were assigned to a trained group ($N = 35$) or a control group ($N = 30$). The multidimensional ELS test protocol (Dejonckere et al., 2001) and the Voice Loading Test (lingWAVES, 2007) were applied in both groups at the study onset and after 4 months. The voice training consisted of 3 hours of indirect training (a theoretical lecture) and 3 hours of direct training (a lecture with exercises). In the small groups (six or eight students) undergoing direct training, they were asked to perform the exercises in front of the class. Very little feedback was given to each student. The training was structured and scripted. More details of this study are given in Timmermans et al. (2011).

It should be made clear that ostentatious results were not expected. The aim was to inform students and to warn them about the risk of voice problems. Nevertheless, several significant differences between the trained and control group were found.

It is now clear that these training sessions made a difference. The fact that the future teachers are clearly told what is good or bad for the voice, how the voice should be used and which techniques need to be used has a limited but important impact. Further research is planned to investigate whether these prevention programmes really protect professionals against future voice problems.

# Warming-up

Another important issue for professional voice users is whether vocal warm-up exercises have an impact on vocal quality. According to Heurer *et al.* (2006), warm-up is important in voice training and prepares the vocal folds and muscles for the demands of the day. A warm-up routine includes muscular strength of motion exercises (useful for relaxation and to heighten the patient's tactile feedback system), phonation and speaking exercises. Vocal warm-up exercises are expected to increase blood flow to the vocal folds and decrease muscle viscosity and perhaps non-muscular tissue viscosity (Milbrath & Solomon, 2003).

The purpose of the study of Van Lierde *et al.* (2010) was to determine the impact of a specific vocal warm-up programme on objective vocal quality using a multiparameter approach (DSI) in female students training to be speech-language pathologists (SLPs). Hypothetically, one can assume that the objective vocal quality will increase after vocal warm-up exercises in future professional voice users compared to the matched control group who receive no warm-up programme. Forty-five female subjects of an experimental subject group (who received 30 minutes of warm-up exercises) were compared with 45 female subjects in the control group. The methodological details are described elsewhere in detail (Van Lierde *et al.*, 2010a).

The main purpose of the vocal warm-up programme is to improve the dynamics of the laryngeal muscles. Exercises were selected both to improve muscle flexibility and also to enhance voice production awareness.

As hypothesised, the results of this study showed significant improvement of the objective vocal quality after a vocal warm-up of 30 minutes. No improvement was measured in the control group after 30 minutes of vocal rest. As the DSI is a weighted variable, small improvements are indicative of vocal quality changes (Wuyts *et al.*, 2000) and it is found to be a sensitive tool for quantifying the effect of various vocal therapy techniques (Van Lierde *et al.*, 2010a). After vocal warm-up the voices of the female students had an overall increased objective vocal quality, increased vocal performance

(with lower intensity and higher frequency capacities) and increased fundamental frequency. Long-term effects and the influence of the content of the
warm-up programme are subjects for further research.

# Effectiveness of Voice Therapy Techniques for Pathological Voices

The overall aim of voice therapy is to improve vocal quality by teaching
patients to use their vocal mechanism more efficiently. The therapist can use
direct therapy techniques (by working on posture, breathing, phonation and
articulation) and indirect approaches (voice counselling) to establish the
most efficient voice. In traditional voice therapy approaches, the patient
relies on auditory, tactual and proprioceptive feedback. Therapy duration in
Europe tends to last quite a long time and most of the vocal therapy techniques employed were not the subject of research experiments regarding efficiency. From 2000 onwards, research started to document the outcome of
vocal performances after using specific well-defined vocal therapy techniques. A few of these techniques are discussed as follows.

## Laryngeal feedback

A relatively new strategy for the treatment of voice disorders is the use
of laryngeal biofeedback. In this approach, an ear, nose and throat (ENT)
specialist and the voice therapist collaborate, while individuals learn how to
change their laryngeal posture or movements by watching their own larynges in real time. The combination of tactual, auditory and proprioceptive
information with visual biofeedback by watching desirable or undesirable
laryngeal behaviour shortens treatment duration, with results evident in a
few sessions (Casper et al., 1981). A rigid or flexible fibre-optic laryngoscope
in combination with video equipment can be used to visualise the larynx.
When effective, the treatment is simple and fast. Van Lierde et al. (2004a)
showed the effectiveness of laryngeal biofeedback treatment in two subjects,
a 14-year-old girl and a 15-year-old boy with hyperkinetic dysphonia.
Objective DSI as well as subjective perceptual evaluation techniques were
used. These patients underwent traditional voice therapy with a frequency
of one to two times a week for 6 months. However, they continued to speak
with a hyperkinetic voice. A video-laryngostroboscopy showed, in both children, a muscle tension pattern (MTP) type I (Rubin et al., 1995), revealing a
gap between the vocal processes. Both patients were selected for laryngeal
biofeedback and showed an improvement in their perceptual voice quality
and an improvement in their DSI scores (from DSI value −0.7 before laryngeal biofeedback to +1.4 after laryngeal biofeedback in one subject, and from
−2.5 before laryngeal biofeedback to −0.6 after laryngeal biofeedback in the

other). The improvement of the objective measures is in agreement with the perceived improvement of voice quality.

## Manual circumlaryngeal treatment

Another relatively new management strategy for the treatment of vocal hyperfunction is manual circumlaryngeal treatment (MCT) or laryngeal manual therapy. The aim of MCT is to alter the state of tight vocal tract muscles and to improve the range of movements of the laryngeal joints (Aronson, 1990). Several techniques can be used, such as soft tissue stretch, articulation of laryngeal joints, muscle energy and counterstrain. Compared with traditional voice therapy, the proprioceptive feedback in laryngeal manual therapy is enhanced. Stages of reducing laryngeal muscle tension have also been described by Aronson (1990), Roy and Leeper (1993), Roy et al. (1997) and Greene and Mathieson (1991). Changes in vocal quality after a MCT programme were analysed by Van Lierde et al. (2004b) in four professional voice users in whom traditional voice therapy had not been successful. Objective (aerodynamic, voice range, acoustic and DSI measurements) as well as subjective (video-laryngostroboscopic and auditory perceptual evaluation) assessment techniques were used in the pre- and post-treatment conditions. The MCT was organised in nine steps within 25 therapeutic sessions, at least once but mostly twice a week. The subjects were instructed to exercise twice daily for 5 minutes at home.

All of the subjects selected for MCT showed improvement in perceptual vocal quality and DSI values. The improvement in the objective acoustic results in this study is in agreement with the perceived improvement of strain, hoarseness and the overall grade of vocal pathology. The use of a mixture of the classic principles of voice therapy with repeated laryngeal manipulation seems to be very helpful and motivating for professional voice users with persistent moderate-to-severe muscle tension dysphonia in this pilot study. None of these patients complained of severe discomfort or side effects during or after the manipulation. The authors speculate that the success of laryngeal manual therapy in these subjects can be ascribed to the increased proprioceptive feedback.

Whether MCT is more effective than another voice treatment technique such as vocalisation with abdominal breath support was another research question. In Belgium, many voice specialists use the direct modification of breathing as the start of symptomatic voice therapy. This treatment approach of respiration combined with vocalisation is used because respiration is one of the three major subsystems responsible for the production of voice. Moreover, several authors conclude, on the one hand, that it is evident that some laryngeal pathologies certainly alter normal respiration, especially in muscle tension dysphonia and, on the other hand, that a better breathing pattern can lead to better phonation.

Based on the results of previous reports, by using MCT as the therapeutic technique, a significant improvement in the objective overall vocal quality can be expected. Ten subjects with a mean age of 58 years with muscle tension dysphonia, increased tension of the laryngeal muscles without evidence of laryngeal lesions or laryngeal neuropathology, were included in this study (Van Lierde et al., 2010b). None of the subjects followed voice therapy. The same assessment protocol as in the above-mentioned studies was used.

The experimental therapy design was as follows: before MCT the treatment technique of vocalisation with abdominal breath support was performed for 45 minutes. The objective voice measurement protocol (as described above) was successively done before and after treatment approach 1 (vocalisation with abdominal breath support) and before and after treatment approach 2 (MCT).

As hypothesised, the results of this study showed significant improvement of the objective vocal quality after MCT. The DSI of the subjects improved from −5.9 to −2 after MCT. The significant improvement in the DSI data after MCT showed that one single treatment approach of 45 minutes using MCT is more effective than a similar time spent on abdominal breathing support associated with voice production. Moreover, this study supports the suggestions of Roy and Leeper (1993) and Roy et al. (1997) that manual MCT should be considered early in the treatment selection process. Aronson (1990) suggested that the chronic posture of the larynx in an elevated position leads to cramping and stiffness of the hyoid-laryngeal musculature. Also in these 10 subjects laryngeal elevation and increased tension of the extrinsic and intrinsic laryngeal muscles was observed, which contributes to the occurrence of muscle tension dysphonia. As Aronson (1990) pointed out, MCT is a direct method to treat laryngeal hyperfunction. A direct decrease in laryngeal tension and an immediate voice improvement can be expected. The treatment technique of abdominal breath support combined with voice production can be considered as an indirect method to decrease the laryngeal tension. Limitations of this study are that the assessment of outcome is limited to objective measures; a perceptual evaluation and a self-rating would have been valuable information. To what extent there exists a cumulative therapy effect by combining the two therapy approaches and to what extent the improvement in vocal quality after MCT can be maintained are subjects for future investigation.

## Long-term outcome

As mentioned above, voice therapy in Belgium tends to last a long time because the reimbursement of voice therapy by health insurance is possible for a period of up to 2 years. A question of interest would be: how long is the efficacy duration of a voice rehabilitation programme on vocal behaviour?

It is unclear to what extent a long period of voice therapy contributes to the long-term outcome.

Van Lierde *et al.* (2007) analysed the long-term outcome in a group of 27 (nine males, 18 females) adult subjects with a hyperfunctional voice disorder. The subjects were assessed after 6.1 years on average after their first traditional broad-based voice therapy programme, including vocal hygiene. All patients underwent the above-described voice assessment protocol.

In the laryngovideostrobscopy, 51% of the subjects still showed pathological laryngological findings. In a number of subjects the situation had even worsened from MTP1 to MTP2, a double or longitudinal gap or even a vocal cyst. The negative evolution of the DSI from −1 to −3.2 is in agreement with this finding. On the other hand, perceptual evaluation by the clinician is slightly better for R (roughness), B (breathiness) and S (strained), but remains identical for G (Grade). The VHI score indicates the rather unimportant psychosocial impact of the voice disorder. The more objective findings and laryngostroboscopic findings indicate a chronic situation for a substantial number of the subjects and an even worse situation for some of them. The perceptual findings confirm an unchanged overall hoarseness (G), while patients themselves are less pessimistic about the impact of their voice disorder. These findings at least modify the conclusions about the short-term outcome studies for voice therapy that are in general very positive.

# References

Aronson, A.E. (1990) *Clinical Voice Disorders: An Interdisciplinary Approach* (3rd edn). New York: Thieme.

Berlinger, S. and Bergin, C. (2005) *How to Use Good Vocal Behaviours in the Classroom: An Instructional Videotape for Teachers*. Delray Beach: Minds i No Limits Inc.

Bovo, R., Galceran, M., Petruccelli, J. and Hatzopoulos, S. (2007) Vocal problems among teachers: Evaluation of a preventive voice program. *Journal of Voice* 21 (6), 705–722.

Casper, J.K., Brewer, D.W. and Conture, E.G. (1981) Speech therapy patient evaluation with the fiberscope. In *Transcripts of 10th Symposium: Care of the Professional Voice* (pp. 136–140). New York: Voice Foundation.

Chan, R.W. (1994) Does the voice improve with vocal hygiene education? A study of some instrumental voice measures in a group of kindergarten teachers. *Journal of Voice* 8, 279–291.

De Bodt, M.S., Jacobson, B., Musschoot, S., Zaman, S., Heylen, L., Mertens, F., Van de Heyning, P.H. and Wuyts, F.L. (2000) De Voice Handicap Index. Een instrument voor het kwantificeren van de psychosociale consequenties van stemstoornissen. *Logopedie* 13, 29–33.

Decoster, W. and Debruyne, F. (1997a) The ageing voice: Changes in fundamental frequency, waveform stability and spectrum. *Acta Otorhinolaryngologica Belgica* 51 (2), 105–112.

Decoster, W. and Debruyne, F. (1997b) Changes in spectral measures and voice-onset time with age: A cross-sectional and a longitudinal study. *Folia Phoniatrica et Logopaedica* 49 (6), 269–280.

Dejonckere, P.H., Bradley, P., Clemente, P., Cornut, G., Crevier-Buchman, L., Friedrich, G., Van de Heyning, P.H., Remacle, G. and Woisard, V. (2001) A basic protocol for functional assessment of voice pathology, especially for investigating the efficacy of (phonosurgical) treatments and evaluating new assessment techniques. *European Archives of Otorhinolaryngology* 258, 77–82.

Duffy, O.M. and Hazlett, D.E. (2004) The impact of preventive voice care programs for training teachers: A longitudinal study. *Journal of Voice* 18, 63–70.

Greene, M.C. and Mathieson, L. (1991) *The Voice and Its Disorders*. London: Whurr Publishers.

Heuer, R.J., Rulnick, R.K., Horman, M., Perez, K.S., Emerich, K.A. and Sataloff, R.T. (2006) Voice therapy. In R.T. Sataloff (ed.) *Vocal Health and Pedagogy. Advanced Assessment and Treatment* (2nd edn; pp. 227–251). San Diego: Plural Publishing.

Hirano, M. (1990) Clinical application of voice tests. In NIDCD (ed.) *Assessment of Speech and Voice Production* (Monograph, 27–28 September; pp. 196–203). Maryland: National Institute on Deafness and Other Communication Disorders.

Kaufman, T.J. and Johnson, T.S. (1991) An exemplary preventative voice program for educators. *Seminars in Speech and Language* 12, 40–48.

lingWAVES (2007) lingWAVES version 2.5 [computer software]. Germany: LingCom GmbH. http://www.wevosys.com/

Milbrath, R.L. and Solomon, N.P. (2003) Do vocal warm-up exercises alleviate vocal fatigue? *Journal of Speech, Language and Hearing Research* 46, 422–436.

Morsomme, D. (2001) Contribution a la determination de parametres subjectifs et objectifs pour l'étude de la voix. PhD dissertation, Catholic University of Louvain (UCL).

Pasa, G., Oates, J. and Dacakis, G. (2007) The relative effectiveness of vocal hygiene training and vocal function exercises in preventing voice disorders in primary school teachers. *Logopedics Phoniatrics Vocology* 32, 128–140.

Roy, N. and Leeper, H.A. (1993) Effects of the manual laryngeal musculoskeletal tension reduction technique as a treatment for functional voice disorders: Perceptual and acoustic measures. *Journal of Voice* 7, 242–249.

Roy, N., Bless, D.M., Heisey, D. and Ford, C.N. (1997) Manual circumlaryngeal therapy for functional dysphonia: An evaluation of short- and long-term treatment outcomes. *Journal of Voice* 11, 321–331.

Roy, N., Weinrich, B., Gray, S.D., Tanner, K., Toledo, S.W., Dove, H., Corbin-Lewis, K. and Stemple, J.C. (2004) Voice amplification versus vocal hygiene instruction for teachers with voice disorders: A treatments outcomes study. *Journal of Speech, Language, and Hearing Research* 45, 625–638.

Rubin, J.S., Sataloff, R.T., Korovin, G.S. and Gould, W.J. (1995) *Diagnosis and Treatment of Voice Disorders*. Tokyo: Igaku-Shoin.

Schneider, B. and Bigenzahn, W. (2005) How we do it: Voice therapy to improve vocal constitution and endurance in female student teachers. *Clinical Otolaryngology* 30, 64–78.

Simberg, S. (2004) Prevalence of vocal symptoms and voice disorders among teacher students and teachers and a model of early intervention. Doctoral thesis, University of Helsinki.

Timmermans, B., De Bodt, M., Wuyts, F., Boudewijns, A., Clement, G., Peeters, A. and Van de Heyning, P. (2002) Poor voice quality in future elite vocal performers and professional voice users. *Journal of Voice* 16 (3), 372–382.

Timmermans, B., De Bodt, M., Wuyts F. and Van de Heyning, P. (2003a) Vocal hygiene in future professional voice users and in professional voice users. *Logopedics Phoniatrics Vocology* 28, 127–132.

Timmermans, B., De Bodt, M., Wuyts, F. and Van de Heyning, P. (2003b) Analysis of a voice training program in future voice professionals. *Journal of Voice* 19 (2), 102–110.

Timmermans, B., De Bodt, M., Wuyts, F. and Van de Heyning, P. (2004a) Training outcome in future professional voice users after eighteen months voice training. *Folia Phoniatrica Logopaedica* 56, 120–129.

Timmermans, B., De Bodt, M., Wuyts, F. and Van de Heyning, P. (2004b) Voice quality change in future professional voice users after nine months voice training. *European Archives of Otolaryngologica* 261 (1), 1–5.

Timmermans, B., Coveliers, Y., Meeus, W., Vandenabeele, F., Van Looy, L. and Wuyts, F.L. (2011) The effect of a short voice training program in future teachers. *Journal of Voice* 25 (4), e191–198.

Van de Heyning, P.H., Remacle, M. and Van Cauwenberghe, P. (1996) Functional assessment of voice disorders. Part II: Research work of the Belgian Study Group on Voice Disorders (BSGVD). *Acta Oto-Rhino-Laryngologica Belgica* 50, 4.

Van Lierde, K.M., Claeys, S., De Bodt, M. and Van Cauwenberge, P. (2004a) Outcome of laryngeal and velopharyngeal biofeedback treatment in children and young adults: A pilot study. *Journal of Voice* 18, 97–106.

Van Lierde, K.M., Deley, S., Bernart, L., De Bodt, M. and Van Cauwenberge, P. (2004b) Outcome of manual voice therapy in four Dutch adults with persistent moderate to severe vocal hyperfunction: A pilot study. *Journal of Voice* 18, 467–474.

Van Lierde, K.M., Claeys, S., De Bodt, M. and van Cauwenberge, P. (2007) Long-term outcome of hyperfunctional voice disorders based on a multiparameter approach. *Journal of Voice* 21 (2), 179–188.

Van Lierde, K., D'haeseleer, E., Baudonck, N., Claeys, S., De Bodt, M. and Behlau, M. (2010a) The impact of vocal warm-up exercises on the objective vocal quality in female students training to be speech language pathologists. *Journal of Voice* 25 (3), e115–121.

Van Lierde, K.M., De Bodt, M., D'haeseleer, E., Wuyts, F. and Claeys, S. (2010b) The treatment of muscle tension dysphonia: A comparison of two treatment techniques by means of an objective multiparameter approach. *Journal of Voice* 24, 294–301.

Wuyts, F.L., De Bodt, M.S., Molenberghs, G., Remacle, M., Heylen, L., Millet, B., Van Lierde, K., Raes, J. and Van de Heyning, P.H. (2000) The Dysphonia Severity Index: An objective measure of vocal quality based on a multiparameter approach. *Journal of Speech, Language, and Hearing Research* 43, 796–809.

# 3 Speech Language Pathology and the Voice Specialist in Brazil: An Overview

## Mara Behlau, Gisele Oliveira, Glaucya Madazio and Rosiane Yamasaki

## Introduction

Brazil is the fifth biggest country in the world, with a population of 186,112,794 people (CIA, 2007). The number of speech language pathologists (SLPs) and audiologists in Brazil totaled 33,400. We estimate that there are approximately 280,000 SLPs in the world; 68% are in the Americas – North, Central and South – with 135,000 in the US and 33,000 in Brazil, placing us in the second-rank position as to the number of professionals in a single country. However, most of these 33,400 colleagues hold only a bachelor's degree, without any further education, with only 5304 specialists, 1200 master's and 507 PhD holders. These professionals are registered at the 'Conselho Federal de Fonoaudiologia – CFFa', the institution responsible for monitoring the practice which accepts the bachelor's level as sufficient to begin practice ('CFFa – Especilização [Specialization]').

The profession is called 'Fonoaudiologia' in Brazilian Portuguese. It was officially recognized as an independent health profession on 9 December 1981 (Law #6965/81), although there are some historical notes indicating the existence of practical professionals working with prophylaxis and speech and writing correction since the 1920s and attention to deaf children as early as 1850.

A 'fonoaudiólogo' is a professional with a full university education in both SLP and Audiology, working in research, prevention, evaluation, habilitation and rehabilitation. According to a recent definition, 'SLP and Audiology is the study of human communication, as far as development, training, disorders and differences are concerned, related to aspects involving peripheral and central hearing, vestibular functions, cognitive functions, oral and written language, speech fluency, voice, oral myology functions and swallowing'

(Conselho de Federal, 2004). Brazil has one national professional board (CFFa) and two scientific societies (the Brazilian Society of SLP and Audiology (SBFa) and the Brazilian Academy of Audiology (ABA)) among other smaller specific and multi-professional associations. The SBFa is the major scientific organization for the profession, and has been organizing national and international congresses since 1989.

There are more than 80 undergraduate programs in the country (4-year duration, full-time), heavily concentrated in the south. Graduate programs are limited to eight at master's and three at PhD level (Fernandes *et al.*, 2010). The objectives of the courses are: to improve the quality of the undergraduate programs; to open up new possibilities for graduate programs with a fair geographical distribution; to ensure the quality of services and wages; to be properly covered by health insurance companies; to widen up action on health and education; to ensure continuing education for SLPs; and to extend the scope of practice with new specialized areas.

There are five traditional specialties: audiology, language, voice, oral myology and public health; and two recently recognized ones: dysphagia and educational SLP. Voice specialization programs have existed since the 1990s and there are currently 10 programs in the country, with a minimum of 500 class hours usually distributed across a one-year period. The oldest active and traditional specialization program in voice has been sponsored by the Center for Voice Studies – Superior Institute in Communication Education (CEV-ISEC) since 1993. A total of 935 SLPs hold the specialization in voice title in the country. The title 'Voice Specialist' has been recognized since 1996 by the national professional board, the CFFa – Especilização.

There are three major sub-areas for the SLP specializing in voice: clinical voice, professional voice and head and neck cancer rehabilitation. However, most specialists generally work in two of these domains (clinical voice and head and neck; or clinical and professional voice).

Undergraduate programs in SLP usually focus primarily on language disorders. Most of them cover only the minimum requirement to practice in the voice area. However, the possibility of working with a combination of health and artistic disciplines makes this area appealing. The most studied professional voice users in Brazil are teachers. A recent review of the last 15 years of Brazilian publications (1994–2008) analyzed a total of 500 publications with at least one SLP as their authors (Dragone *et al.*, 2010). The results showed that the majority of the studies were related to vocal assessment (86%), which was the core of the Brazilian research on teachers' voice. Treatment outcome evaluations are emphasized in recent publications (6.2%), and this may reflect a change of focus that can aid understanding of the complex use of voice in teaching and guide future SLP and governmental actions.

Professional voice is one of the most developed voice subspecialties and recently the Department of Voice of the SBFa (Oliveira *et al.*, 2008) issued a video CD with a compilation of the contributions in the area, particularly considering the following aspects: teachers' voice, call center operators, voice-overs, television and radio broadcasters, acting voice, classical and popular singers, clergy, and several occupations with a vocal load, such as brokers, lawyers and businessmen. Moreover, the 28 existing municipal and state laws were presented to give an overview of the legal aspects related to voice as an occupational risk. A current trend is the Corporate SLP focus on communicative competence (speech and listening dimensions, verbal and non-verbal information), within a larger scope than working specifically with voice.

## World Voice Day

World Voice Day (16 April) was established in 1999 with the main goal of increasing public awareness of the importance of voice and alertness to voice problems. The event first started in Brazil in 1999 as the Brazilian National Voice Day. It was the result of a mixed initiative by physicians, SPL and singing teachers belonging to the former association 'Sociedade Brasileira de Laringologia e Voz – SBLV' (Brazilian Society of Laryngology and Voice).

This initiative was followed by other countries, such as Argentina and Portugal, and the Brazilian National Voice Day became the International Voice Day. In the United States, the American Academy of Otolaryngology – Head and Neck Surgery officially recognized this celebration in 2002 and in that year the event was given the name 'World Voice Day' (Švec & Behlau, 2007).

## Main Aspects of Voice Evaluation and Treatment

Dysphonia is any deviation that may restrain natural voice expression (Behlau & Pontes, 1995) and produce a negative self-perceived impact. Since voice is a multidimensional phenomenon, its evaluation must necessarily be multidimensional and should include instruments of perceptual, behavioral, acoustic and visual analysis and self-evaluation protocols. Voice therapy in Brazil is administered by SLPs, preferably specializing in voice, which requires a unique combination of personal characteristics and specific scientific knowledge from the clinician.

There are many challenges that SLPs specializing in voice encounter when trying to assess and treat clients with an optimal practice attitude. From the clinical stance, the broad diagnostic diversity presents itself as a major problem. Although the voice area has evolved from a more abstract and artistic nature into a more structured scientific standpoint, there is still a long way to go in order to routinely use practice-based evidence interventions. The management of a voice patient requires a close partnership between the physician (in Brazil, an otorhinolaryngologist) and the voice clinician in order to properly deal with clinical needs. The essential aspects usually present in almost any scientific discussion in Brazil regarding voice evaluation are: complaints and history of dysphonia, role of vocal behavior on the etiology of the problem, normalcy of voice, vocal parameters, auditory-perceptual and acoustic analysis of voice, self-assessment protocols, body-voice integration, voice-personality equilibrium, environmental factors, and correlation between auditory-visual-acoustic data. As far as voice rehabilitation is concerned, clinicians face challenges such as the utilization of the best available evidence, the decision to administer programmatic or custom-made therapy, and the selection of approaches and therapeutic regimen.

This chapter will highlight the perceptual and acoustic analysis of voice and self-assessment protocols used in voice evaluation. The Brazilian tradition of treatments and therapeutic regimen will also be discussed.

## Evaluation perspective

### Auditory-perceptual analysis of the voice

The basis of the vocal clinical evaluation is an auditory-perceptual analysis performed by means of standardized protocols. However, an average Brazilian clinician still uses descriptive terms and isolated parameters.

There are a wide range of perceptual protocols available, from which we may draw attention to the GRBAS scale and some variants of it (Hirano, 1985; Pinho & Pontes, 2002), the Voice Profile Analysis (VPA; Laver, 1980) and, more recently, the Brazilian version of CAPE-V (Behlau, 2004; Kempster et al., 2009). Experience with the Brazilian CAPE-V seems to suggest that the usefulness of this protocol is somewhat free of cultural bias. The Brazilian CAPE-V uses the most common vocal qualities: roughness, breathiness and strain (Oates, 2009).

This kind of evaluation allows us to distinguish the characterization of vocal quality and the quantification of vocal deviation to a given voice stimulus. The use of a patterned classification system to categorize normal and disordered voices is important in clinical practice and is a methodological challenge.

The normalcy of voice is a common issue for discussion. Difficulties are related to the nature of human perception and to a variable cultural influence (Kreiman et al., 2007; Oates, 2009; Patel & Shrivastav, 2007). Vocal quality varies across different cultures, languages and communities. On what point on a rating scale, e.g. a visual analog scale such as the one used in the CAPE-V, can normal voice be differentiated from abnormal voice? Simberg et al. (2000) have established a limit of 34 points (34 mm) on a 100-point visual analog scale (VAS) as the screening threshold. A Brazilian reproduction of this study with 211 voice samples from adults with and without vocal complaints yields a very close limit of 35.5 points (Yamasaki et al., 2008). A receiver operating characteristic (ROC) curve produced three cut-off values

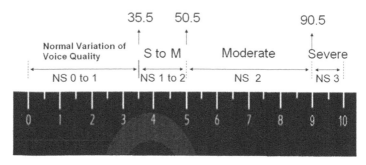

**Figure 3.1** Cut-off values for the Brazilian visual analog scale (VAS) study. S to M, slight to moderate deviation

with large areas (Figure 3.1): 35.5 mm for voice within normal variability of vocal quality and mild deviations (efficiency = 0.918); 50.5 mm for moderate deviations (efficiency = 0.948); and 90.5 mm for severe deviations (efficiency = 0.970). The use of the term normal variation of voice quality (NVVQ) is an attempt to envisage the acceptable variations and can express either the manifestation of vocal style, preference of voice use, professional characterization, or a vocal problem on a mild level. It is interesting to note that the cut-off point for the same overall evaluation using the CAPE-V by American listeners was 11 mm.

## Acoustic analysis of the voice

The use of acoustic analysis in voice evaluation is not meant to replace perceptual analysis. Using acoustics in the voice clinic allows one to record, quantify and produce a baseline for treatment follow-up.

In the past, the use of acoustic resources was limited to university and hospital centers, due to the expense involved in their development and acquisition. A partnership between the Centre for Voice (CEV – a research institute), and CTS Informatica (a computer development company) was established in 2002 to develop user-friendly and low-cost products for SLPs. A series of five programs have been created: VOXMETRIA, FONOVIEW, FONOTOOLS, VOXGAMES and VOCALGRAMA. All software is available in Portuguese, English, Spanish and Korean, except VOCALGRAMA, the newest one, which is still only offered in Portuguese.

VOXMETRIA is software for voice clinical evaluation which provides fast and dynamic acoustic assessment and is an educational resource for the clinician and patient. It produces a phonatory deviation diagram (PDD) that locates the voice deviation and treatment progress in a graph. The PDD is based on four acoustic measurements, three of them related to signal irregularities and one related to the glottal-to-noise excitation ratio (GNE). A recent study (Madazio & Behlau, 2010) showed that all normal voices were placed in the inferior left quadrant (normal area) of the PDD, 45% of rough voices were found in the inferior right quadrant, 52.6% of breathy voices in the superior right quadrant, and 54.3% of tense voices in the inferior left quadrant, with statistically significant differences. In the inferior left quadrant, 93.8% of dysphonic voices with mild deviation and 72.7% with moderate deviation were found. Voices with a severe degree of deviation were distributed in the inferior right and both superior quadrants, with the latter ones containing the most deviant voices and 80% of extremely deviated voices. Thus, the PDD proves to be an instrument that is able to discriminate normal from dysphonic voices and the distribution is related to the type and degree of voice deviation (Figure 3.2).

FONOVIEW was developed to optimize the use of real-time spectrographic analysis in the voice clinic. It is a user-friendly software and it allows the development of the visual-vocal and audio-vocal monitoring of a number of voice and speech parameters. In order to determine the relationship between perceptual and acoustic data, 184 Brazilian voice samples classified as mainly rough, breathy and strained were spectrographically analyzed (FONOVIEW, CTS Informatica) to determine the most important visual characteristics on the spectrographic display (Behlau & Leão, 2009). Rough voices were characterized by frequency bifurcation and noise at low frequencies, breathy voices by noise at both high and low frequencies, and strained voices by instability and rich series of harmonics. This information is not only helpful in clinical practice but also considered complementary to perceptual evaluation.

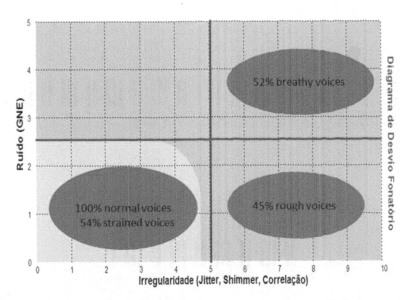

**Figure 3.2** Distribution of voice types on the phonatory deviation diagram, with irregularity on the horizontal axis (jitter, shimmer and correlation) and noise on the vertical axis (Glottic to Noise Excitation – GNE)

The development of FONOTOOLS was based on the need for a simple resource to employ the auditory method on the improvement and rehabilitation of dysphonia. Auditory control seems to be crucial for human vocalization. FONOTOOLS is a low-cost application that encompasses diverse modes of voice hearing manipulation and it allows the visualization and storage of voice recordings. The operation modes are amplification, delay, frequency change, inversion, masking, loop and rhythm. This system can be used as an aid to rehabilitation in many dysphonia cases, such as Parkinson's disease (Coutinho *et al.*, 2009).

VOCALGRAMA was developed to provide voice and speech range profiles, allowing the assessment of speaking and singing adjustments. This software is an instrument that provides data on voice production in different frequencies and intensities. It is an easy-to-use tool that allows the identification of healthy and dysphonic voices and provides treatment follow-up by comparing clients' registers and by producing simple graphs. The speech range profile is a promising strategy for evaluating, educating and rehabilitating a patient. A recent study showed a graph of a stable oval-like shape for normal voices, an enlarged and scattered distribution for behavioral dysphonia (false broad area), and a constricted area for neurological cases, respectively (Figure 3.3; Behlau *et al.*, 2010; Moraes & Behlau, 2010).

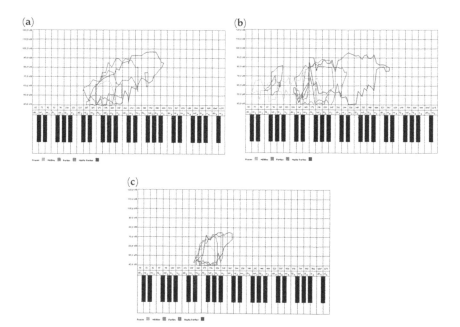

**Figure 3.3** VOCALGRAMA shape for: (a) normal voices (oval distribution); (b) behavioral dysphonia (enlarged/scattered distribution); (c) neurological dysphonia (constricted distribution)

Besides these evaluative software programs, the partnership has also developed VOXGAMES, 25-game software for pediatric voice therapy to provide control over the following aspects: loudness, pitch, phonation time, voice and unvoiced phonemes, and sound-silence status.

## Self-assessment protocols

In recent decades, rehabilitation focuses have shifted from the perspective of the clinician to that of the patient. This concept probably represents one of the most important contributions to the evaluation and treatment process of any disease. A patient's self-assessment of his/her vocal problem and the analysis of the results of a treatment are useful means to ascertain the effectiveness of an intervention. Psychometric instruments use the questionnaire format as the most common tool used to perform this task. Many of these questionnaires were originally developed in English. In case these instruments are adopted for use in other languages, they will need to be translated, adapted and their measuring properties subjected to psychometric tests (Ciconelli et al., 1999; Guillemin et al., 1993). The three most commonly used self-assessment protocols are the Voice-Related Quality of Life (Hogikyan & Sethuraman, 1999), Voice Handicap Index (Jacobson et al., 1997) and the Voice Activity and Participation Profile (Ma & Yiu, 2001). All protocols were validated in Brazilian Portuguese based on the guidelines set by the Scientific Advisory Committee of the Medical Outcomes Trust (SAC), and each of them has its own advantages and limitations.

Coping strategy is considered an important concept in the health area and in the context of quality of life. It is deeply associated with the regulation of emotions during a stressful period. However, there is no consensus about which strategies are more adequate or how a specific type of coping strategy might contribute to solving a problem or alleviating emotional stress. When the mediating role of a coping strategy is taken into consideration (Folkman, 1984; Folkman & Lazarus, 1985; Folkman et al., 1986), it becomes easier to understand the diversity of treatment outcomes of a voice problem, and the importance of addressing this issue adequately during the intervention process, since the expected result is that the individual will adapt effectively to the situation. SLPs should help patients to identify strategies they can use to cope with their voice disorders and to change those strategies that do not promote adaptation (Meulenbroek & de Jong, 2010; Van Opstal, 2010). One of the early studies on coping with dysphonia (Epstein, 1999) investigated coping strategies used by individuals with spasmodic dysphonia and with muscle tension dysphonia. The findings of this study led to the development of a self-report questionnaire that assesses coping with voice disorders – the Voice Disability Coping Questionnaire (VDCQ; Epstein et al., 2009). Another study used the VDCQ in a Brazilian population to explore the coping strategies of individuals with and without vocal complaints and to examine the relationships between the type of coping and the vocal complaint, vocal symptoms, vocal self-assessment, perceptual analysis and states of depression, anxiety, aspects related to self-esteem, and locus of control (Oliveira et al., 2010). These findings indicated that people with vocal complaints used a variety of coping strategies – problem-focused ones in particular – to deal with their voice problems.

## Treatment aspects

Voice therapy has long been a tradition in Brazil. The two main pioneer clinicians are from Rio de Janeiro city – Professor Edmée Brandi Melo and Professor Maria da Gloria Beutenmuller. Mello (1972) developed the Brandi Scales for voice evaluation and the Inductive Progressive Method for dysphonia treatment, aiming to help the speakers reformulate their vocal schema on their own. Beutenmuller developed the Spatial Directional Method (Beuttenmuller & Laport, 1974) associating vocal to body expression using a rhythm-based approach. This so-called 'global shape of the word' has been employed by Brazilian professional voice users, in drama and television broadcasting settings.

The voice disorders identification, diagnosis and treatment method that we use is based on a global approach (Behlau & Pontes, 1995). The global approach corresponds to an eclectic process for dysphonia rehabilitation. This approach takes into consideration the different phonatory apparatus subsystems, the individual's biological, psychological and emotional dimensions, and integrates the individual's communication relationships with the world.

The global approach for vocal rehabilitation involves analyzing its causes, identifying the deviated vocal parameters, defining the phonatory and non-phonatory laryngeal configurations, as well as considering the emotional history, the dysphonia vocal psychodynamics and the different communication roles of the individual. Voice intervention focuses directly on the production of a more adequate and efficient vocal quality, by means of therapeutic processes that provide an immediate vocal change.

The global approach encompasses seven general methods for voice rehabilitation (Behlau, 2005): (1) Body Method; (2) Phonoarticulatory Organs Method; (3) Auditory Method; (4) Speech Method; (5) Facilitating Sounds Method; (6) Phonatory Competence Method; and (7) Voice Activation Method. The Body Method consists of several techniques using either global or specific body movements and posture to produce a better voice output. The Phonoarticulatory Organs Method employs a number of techniques that manipulate the tongue, mouth and pharynx, in order to improve voice production. The Auditory Method is based on the use of the transformed listening (e.g. amplification, masking, loop, delay auditory feedback and/or vocal pacing using FONOTOOLS (CTS Informatica, Brazil) of one's own voice to achieve easier phonation. The Speech Method uses varied speech production to interact with sound source and resonance. The Facilitating Sounds Method encompasses different selected sounds, such as: nasal sounds; tongue and lips vibration sounds; and fricative, plosive, basal and hyper-high-pitch production for specific purposes. The Phonatory Competence Method is based on improving the laryngeal valve at the glottic or supraglottic level by means of muscle adjustments. The Voice Activation Method uses a range of techniques to facilitate phonation at the glottic level or an alternative voice production.

Selection for therapy method takes into consideration medical diagnosis, vocal evaluation, therapeutic purpose, prognosis, short- or long-term results, the known efficiency of the selected technique, personality traits of the patient and the experience of the clinician in using the specific technique. Therefore, a customized approach to cater for the needs of the patient is important.

The frequency of the intervention program should also be carefully considered. If there is a specific and urgent need for voice use, such as in the case of a professional voice user who needs to be on stage, an intensive program is a better option than weekly therapy. On the other hand, for behavioral-based dysphonias, a regular basis regimen offers a more stable result. The frequency of sessions and/or exercises is still unclear and relies basically on the clinician's experience. There is not enough data available on the time of execution, resting period between series, number of repetitions, frequency and strength of performance. Many questions regarding the physiology of vocal exercises need to be scientifically addressed. Immediate vocal changes are often easy to achieve but long-term maintenance is not.

Brazilian citizens have been using private health services as an alternative to public health services for decades. On 7 June 2009, a new Normative Resolution (#211 law #9.656/98) regarding the extension of SLP services for all health insurance plan holders began. This resolution would benefit approximately 44 million Brazilians who subscribed to health plans from 1 January 1999. To date, the health insurance companies have to provide Brazilians with at least 24 sessions per year, rather than only six as in the past.

Close collaboration between physicians and SLPs in Brazil helps us bring about a better understanding of voice disorders and the approaches that can be used to assess and treat them. Voice is multidimensional and it requires contributions from those with varied expertise.

# References

Behlau, M. (2004) Consensus auditory-perceptual evaluation of voice (CAPE-V), ASHA 2003. *Revista da Sociedade Brasileira de Fonoaudiologia* 9 (3), 187–189.

Behlau, M. (2005) *Voz – O livro do especialista* (Vol. 2). Rio de Janeiro: Revinter.

Behlau, M. and Leão, S. (2009) Spectrographic analysis of voice classified as rough, breathy and strained. Paper presented at the 7th European CPLOL Congress Proceedings, Slovenia.

Behlau, M. and Pontes, P. (1995) *Avaliação e tratamento das disfonias*. São Paulo: Lovise.

Behlau, M., Moraes, M. and Oliveira, G. (2010) Low cost software solutions for clinical voice. Paper presented at the 28th World Congress of the International Association of Logopedics and Phoniatrics, 22–26 August, Athens.

Beuttenmuller, M.G. and Laport, N. (1974) *Expressão vocal e expressão corporal*. Rio de Janeiro: Forense-Universitária.

CFFa – Especilização (Specialization), accessed 22 July 2010. http://www.fonoaudiologia.com/informa/etica/

CIA (2007) *The World Factbook 2005*. Online document: https://www.cia.gov/library/publications/download/download-2005/

Ciconelli, R.M., Ferraz, M.B., Santos, W., Meinão, I. and Quaresma, M.R. (1999) Tradução para a língua portuguesa e validação do questionário genérico de avaliação de qualidade de vida SF-36 (Brasil SF-36). *Revista Brasileira de Reumatologia* 39 (3), 143–150.

Conselho de Federal (2004) *Code of Ethics*, accessed 5 March 2012. http://www.fonoaudiologia.org.br/paginas_internas/pdf/codeport.pdf

Coutinho, S.B., Diaféria, G., Oliveira, G. and Behlau, M. (2009) Voz e fala de Parkinsonianos durante situações de amplificação, atraso e mascaramento. *Pró-Fono Revista de Atualização Científica* 21, 219–224.

Dragone, M.L.S., Ferreira, L.P., Giannini, S.P.P., Simões-Zenari, M., Vieira, V.P. and Behlau, M. (2010) Voz do professor: uma revisão de 15 anos de contribuição fonoaudiológica Teachers' voice: A review of 15 years of SLP contribution. *Revista da Sociedade Brasileira de Fonoaudiologia* 15 (2), 289–296.

Epstein, R. (1999) The impact of botulinum toxin injections in adductor spasmodic dysphonia: A cross-sectional and longitudinal study. Unpublished doctoral thesis, University of London.

Epstein, R., Hirani, S.P., Stygall, J. and Newman, S.P. (2009) How do individuals cope with voice disorders? Introducing the Voice Disability Coping Questionnaire. *Journal of Voice* 23 (2), 209–217.

Fernandes, F.D.M., de Andrade, C.R.F., Befi-Lopes, D.M., Wertzner, H.F. and Limongi, S.C.O. (2010) Emerging issues concerning the education of speech and language pathologists and audiologists in Brazil and South America. *Folia Phoniatrica et Logopaedica* 62, 223–227.

Folkman, S. (1984) Personal control and stress and coping processes: A theoretical analysis. *Journal of Personality and Social Psychology* 46 (4), 839–852.

Folkman, S. and Lazarus, R.S. (1985) If it changes it must be a process: Study of emotion and coping during three stages of a college examination. *Journal of Personality and Social Psychology* 48 (1), 150–170.

Folkman, S., Lazarus, R.S., Dunkel-Schetter, C., DeLongis, A. and Gruen, R.J. (1986) Dynamics of a stressful encounter: Cognitive appraisal, coping, and encounter outcomes. *Journal of Personality and Social Psychology* 50 (5), 992–1003.

Guillemin, F., Bombardier, C. and Beaton, D. (1993) Cross-cultural adaptation of health-related quality of life measures: Literature review and proposed guidelines. *Journal of Clinical Epidemiology* 46 (12), 1417–1432.

Hirano, M. (1985) *Clinical Examination of Voice*. New York: Springer-Verlag.

Hogikyan, N.D. and Sethuraman, G. (1999) Validation of an instrument to measure voice-related quality of life (V-RQOL). *Journal of Voice* 13 (4), 557–569.

Jacobson, B.H., Johnson, A., Grywalski, C., Silbergleit, A., Jacobson, G., Benninger, M.S., *et al.* (1997) The Voice Handicap Index (VHI): Development and validation. *American Journal of Speech-Language Pathology* 6, 66–70.

Kempster, G.B., Gerratt, B.R., Verdolini Abbott, K., Barkmeier-Kraemer, J. and Hillman, R.E. (2009) Consensus auditory-perceptual evaluation of voice: Development of a standardized clinical protocol. *American Journal of Speech-Language-Hearing Association* 18, 124–132.

Kreiman, J., Gerratt, B.R. and Ito, M. (2007) When and why listeners disagree in voice quality assessment tasks. *Journal of Acoustic Society of America* 122 (4), 2354–2364.

Laver, J. (1980) *The Phonetic Description of Voice Quality* (Cambridge Studies in Linguistics, Vol. 31). London: Cambridge University Press.

Ma, E.P-M. and Yiu, E.M-L. (2001) Voice Activity and Participation Profile: Assessing the impact of voice disorders on daily activities. *Journal of Speech, Language, and Hearing Research* 44, 511–524.

Madazio, G. and Behlau, M. (2010) Phonatory deviation diagram in voice clinic. Paper presented at the 28th World Congress of the International Association of Logopedics and Phoniatrics (IALP) Proceedings, Athens.

Mello, E.B.S. (1972) *Educação da voz falada: Exercícios originais da autora*. Rio de Janeiro: Edições Gernasa.

Meulenbroek, L.F.P. and de Jong, F.I.C.R.S. (2010) Trainee experience in relation to voice handicap, general coping and psychosomatic well-being in female student teachers: A descriptive study. *Folia Phoniatrica et Logopaedica* 62, 47–54.

Moraes, M. and Behlau, M. (2010) Voice (VRP) and Speech Range Profile (SRP) in the voice clinic. Paper presented at the 28th World Congress of the International Association of Logopedics and Phoniatrics, Athens.

Oates, J. (2009) Auditory-perceptual evaluation of disordered voice quality – pros, cons and future directions. *Folia Phoniatrica et Logopaedica* 61, 49–56.

Oliveira, G., Epstein, R., Hirani, S., Yagizi, L. and Behlau, M. (2010) *Coping strategies in voice disorders*. Paper presented at the 28th World Congress of the International Association of Logopedics and Phoniatrics, 22–26 August, Athens.

Oliveira, I.B., Almeida, A.A. and Raize, T. (2008) Voz profissional. Produção científica da fonoaudiologia brasileira. *Revista da Sociedade Brasileira de Fonoaudiologia (suppl)* [CD-ROM].

Patel, S. and Shrivastav, R. (2007) Perception of dysphonic vocal quality: Some thoughts and research update. *Voice and Voice Disorders* 17 (2), 3–6.

Pinho, S.R.M. and Pontes, P.A.L. (2002) Escala de avaliação perceptiva da fonte glótica: RASAT. *Vox Brasilis* 3 (1), 11–13.

Simberg, S., Laine, A., Sala, E. and Rönnemaa, A.-M. (2000) Prevalence of voice disorders among future teachers. *Journal of Voice* 14 (2), 231–235.

Švec, J.G. and Behlau, M. (2007) April 16th: The World Voice Day. *Folia Phoniatrica et Logopaedica* 59 (2), 53–54.

Van Opstal, M.J.M.C. (2010) A systematic, holistic and integrative process of self-control for voicing with optimal coping effects in teachers. A process of change – an expert's opinion. *Folia Phoniatrica et Logopaedica* 62 (1–2), 71–85.

Yamasaki, R., Leão, S.H.S., Madazio, G., Padovani, M., Azevedo, R. and Behlau, M. (2008) Correspondência entre Escala Analógico-Visual e a Escala Numérica na Avaliação Perceptivo-Auditiva de Vozes. Paper presented at the XVI Congresso Brasileiro de Fonoaudiologia, Campos de Jordão, Sao Paulo.

# 4 Current Issues in Voice Assessment and Intervention in China

## Wen Xu and Demin Han

## Introduction

The clinical examination of voice disorders involves a morphological appraisal of the larynx, vocal function evaluations (e.g. aerodynamic measures, voice range profile), voice quality analysis (acoustic and auditory-perceptual measures), vocal fold vibration characteristics and electrophysiological assessments. With the rapid developments in modern laryngology, a variety of clinical assessment tools have been developed and used widely. In China, these assessments are generally carried out by physicians as the speech pathology/therapy profession does not exist.

In China, indirect laryngoscopy is the first line of clinical assessment used in the screening of general ear, nose and throat (ENT) problems. Flexible laryngoscopy is a popular assessment tool used in many hospitals in China for examining patients with nasal, pharyngeal or laryngeal disorders. Stroboscopy, however, is only found in a few specialized large voice centers across the nation. Auditory-perceptual voice assessment, such as the GRBAS (Grade, Roughness, Breathiness, Asthenia, Strain) scale (Hirano, 1981), is becoming less popular now. Instead, acoustic measurement, as an objective tool, is being used predominately in many voice centers in China. Radiographic evaluation using plain X-ray, CT scan or Magnetic Resonance Imaging (MRI) for evaluating pharyngolaryngeal structures is also commonly used. Assessment of laryngo-esophageal reflux using pH monitoring is a common practice among many voice specialists.

The authors of this chapter work at one of the largest voice centers in China (Voice Center, Beijing Tongren Hospital, Capital Medical University). Videolaryngostroboscopy and vocal function evaluations have been part of the standard diagnostic test protocol for dysphonic patients since 1999. Perceptual assessment using the GRBAS scale, acoustic analysis including the fundamental frequency, jitter, shimmer and noise-to-harmonic ratio, aerodynamic measure of maximum phonation time (MPT), and stroboscopic analysis covering the areas of vocal fold shape, overall glottal closure, mucosal wave normality and supraglottic configuration are the standard assessment procedures for dysphonic patients. The authors also try to investigate the diagnostic potential of ultrasound in cases of pediatric vocal fold paralysis (Wang *et al.*, 2011).

More recently, two areas of clinical voice assessment have gained much attention in clinical practice in China: (1) voice-related quality of life; and (2) laryngeal electromyography. Voice specialists have put more emphasis on taking a holistic approach by taking into account the patients' own perspective of how voice problems affect their quality of life. Voice-related quality of life has become part of the assessment protocol in some major hospitals (Xu *et al.*, 2010). Laryngeal electromyography has also been used extensively by voice specialists in diagnosing neuromuscular-related dysphonia. This chapter will discuss these two developments in China.

## Development and Application of the Chinese Version of the Voice Handicap Index

Voice specialists in China recognize the importance of taking into consideration patients' own personal perceptions of the impact of dysphonia on their quality of life. This has led to the development of a clinical tool so that this area can be included in the routine clinical voice assessment (Li *et al.*, 2009). Some of the available tools reported in the literature include the Voice Handicap Index (VHI), the Voice-Related Quality of Life (V-RQOL) measure (Hogikyan & Sethuraman, 1999), the Voice Outcome Survey and the Voice Symptom Scale (VoiSS; Deary *et al.*, 2003). The VHI was developed in 1997 by Jacobson and colleagues. A number of studies have reported that the VHI is clinically useful for evaluating the effectiveness of voice therapies. To date, the VHI questionnaire has been translated and adapted into Portuguese (Guimarães & Abberton, 2004), Dutch (Hakkesteegt *et al.*, 2006), Hebrew (Amir *et al.*, 2006) and Chinese (Xu *et al.*, 2008). Studies by Hsiung *et al.* (2003) and Lam *et al.* (2006) reported the application of the VHI in Taiwan (Taiwanese) and Hong Kong (Cantonese) Chinese populations respectively. However, the reliability and validity of the Chinese VHI were not addressed in the study by Hsiung *et al.* (2003), while the VHI reported by Lam *et al.* (2006) is only useful for the Cantonese dialect used in Hong Kong. A Mandarin Chinese version of the VHI was therefore developed in China, which took into account the specific cultural needs of Mainland Chinese (see Appendix 4.1). The validation procedure was reported by Xu *et al.* (2010). The level of reliability and internal consistency is similar to other language versions of the VHI.

The Mandarin version of the VHI demonstrated construct validity (Xu et al., 2008, 2010). It is able to discriminate between different types of voice disorders. In our study, the total VHI scores and subscale scores were significantly higher for the dysphonic groups than for the control group, and there was a significant difference among different types of voice disorders ($P < 0.01$). Patients with spasmodic dysphonia showed the highest VHI score. This was followed by unilateral vocal fold paralysis, functional dysphonia, sulcus vocalis, benign and malignant tumor of vocal fold, benign vocal fold disorders (vocal fold cyst, Reinke's edema, vocal fold polyp, vocal nodule) and chronic laryngitis. The emotional subscale score was highest in the spasmodic dysphonia population, followed by functional dysphonia. This suggested that emotional and psychological factors impact greatly on the quality of life of these patients. Patients with specifically high emotional subscale scores may require additional help from a psychologist before or after laryngological treatment in order to achieve a sustainable successful outcome. In the other patient groups, the physical scores were higher than the functional and emotional scores. In addition, treatment also leads to statistically significant improvement in the VHI scores ($P < 0.05$).

Recently, the Mandarin version of the VHI has been used to evaluate the effectiveness of phonosurgery (Xu et al., 2009a) and voice therapy (Duan et al., 2010). The VHI scores, together with the perceptual voice quality and vocal functions, improved significantly following surgery. Duan et al. (2010) reported the efficacy of a voice training program. They found that the treatment group showed significant improvement in their VHI scores while the control group showed no significant changes over time.

We have recently investigated the reliability and validity of a short version of the Mandarin VHI (Li et al., 2012). The study compared the sensitivity of three short versions of VHI: VHI-7, VHI-10 and VHI-13. Preliminary results showed that VHI-10 and VHI-13 demonstrated good reliability and validity(see Appendix 4.2). We proposed that VHI-10 would be the best choice out of the three (cf. Rosen et al., 2004).

# Laryngeal Electromyography in the Diagnosis of Laryngeal Neuromuscular Disorders

Laryngeal electromyography (LEMG) has been used for the study of laryngeal nerve and muscle functions since the late 1950s (Buchthal, 1959; Faaborg-Andersen & Buchthal, 1956). Voice specialists have since then realized the usefulness of LEMG in assessing and diagnosing neurological dysphonia (Mu & Yang, 1991; Xu et al., 2007). LEMG instruments generally include electrodes, amplifiers, a display system, a loudspeaker and a set of data storage devices. Since 2003 our Voice Center has been conducting research on laryngeal neuromuscular disorders by using LEMG. We have studied the electrophysiology of vocal fold immobility (Xu *et al.*, 2007, 2012) and the electrophysiological char-acteristics of the larynx in myasthenia gravis (Xu *et al.*, 2009b).

## Laryngeal electromyography set-up

The two- and four-channel Nicolet Vikingquest Electromyographic sys-tem (Nicolet Biomedical, Madison, WS) is commonly used in voice clinics in China. In our center, one of the channels is connected with the EMG elec-trodes and another is connected to a microphone for recording acoustic sig-nals synchronously. This allows comparison between the muscle activities and phonation. In an LEMG procedure, different electrode types (surface electrode or needle electrode) have been used to record muscle or nerve elec-trophysiological activities (Hillel, 2001; Jacobs & Finkel, 2002; Koufman *et al.*, 2001; Sataloff *et al.*, 2004, 2010; Xu *et al.*, 2007; Yin *et al.*, 1997). Needle electrodes are more precise and are more appropriate for laryngeal examina-tion. Hence, they are used as standard practice in our center. The choice of appropriate needle electrodes (concentric needle electrodes, bipolar concen-tric needle electrodes, monopolar needle electrodes, hooked wire electrodes or single-fiber electrodes) varies and depends on the type of clinical data required for analysis (Jacobs & Finkel, 2002; Koufman *et al.*, 2001; Sataloff *et al.*, 2004, 2010; Yin *et al.*, 1997). Concentric needle electrodes are preferred as the optimal choice for LEMG study (Jacobs & Finkel, 2002; Xu *et al.*, 2007; Yin *et al.*, 1997). Although single-fiber electromyography (SFEMG) is useful in the evaluation of neuromuscular transmission disorders and the assess-ment of motor unit morphology, using this type of electrode specifically requires the skills of the examiner and the cooperation of the patient. SFEMG is therefore not commonly used for laryngeal diagnosis in China.

In our practice, LEMG data are evaluated by both laryngologists and neurologists. During routine LEMG examination, four types of EMG activi-ties are recorded: needle insertional potentials, nerve spontaneous potentials, motor unit potentials and recruitment potentials.

Concentric needle electrodes are placed percutaneously into the follow-ing muscles: the thyroarytenoid (TA) muscle, the posterior cricoarytenoid (PCA) muscle and the cricothyroid (CT) muscle. Local topical anesthetics are generally not necessary, and may only be useful for recording the activi-ties of the PCA muscle. It is recommended that 1 ml of 0.5% tetracaine hydrochloride be used through the CT membrane. The accuracy of needle placement is confirmed by checking the insertional potential activity during the procedure, the anatomic landmarks used in needle insertion and the relationship of the specific muscles when undergoing phonatory and respira-tory tasks.

Although nerve conduction examination is important in determining the intactness of the neuromuscular system, most voice clinics in China do not routinely include this as a standard LEMG procedure because the nerve conduction examination in the larynx is relatively difficult. Nevertheless, from our observations, laryngeal nerve conduction examination (evoked LEMG) is very useful in identifying and localizing the sites and severity of laryngeal nerve lesions. It can examine the electrical activities of the laryngeal muscles supplied by the specific laryngeal nerve that is stimulated during the examination procedure. Evoked LEMG is performed with monopolar needle electrodes that stimulate the external branch of the superior laryngeal nerve and the recurrent laryngeal nerve. The stimulus intensity used is usually between 6.0 and 24.0 mA. The recording electrode is inserted into the CT muscle to measure the superior laryngeal nerve, and into the TA or PCA muscle to measure the recurrent laryngeal nerve. The amplitudes, latency, duration and waveforms of the response potentials from the CT, TA and PCA muscle are evaluated. It has been suggested that the amplitude of evoked LEMG potentials relates to the function of the axon of the nerve, whereas the latency of the evoked potentials reflects the function of the medulla of the nerve (Kimaid *et al.*, 2004). Thus, these two measures are useful indicators of the severity of the neuropathic laryngeal injury.

## Diagnosis of vocal fold immobility using LEMG

Vocal fold immobility may have multiple causes, including nerve damage, mechanical cricoarytenoid joint fixation, neuromuscular joint disorders or tumor infiltration. It is often difficult to identify the cause of vocal fold immobility solely by clinical examination. Our previous study (Xu *et al.*, 2007) showed that 80% of subjects (87 out of 110) with vocal fold immobility (97 unilateral and 13 bilateral) were identified as having neuropathic laryngeal injuries by the LEMG. More than half of these 87 subjects would not have been identified with neuropathic laryngeal injuries merely by medical history and physical examination. The LEMG also provided information on the severity of the injuries. Increased latent period has been found to be a unique characteristic for diagnosing recurrent laryngeal nerve injury. The evoked potentials can be used to estimate the severity of the impairment.

Signs of re-innervation can be determined from the motor unit potentials, when larger amplitudes are firing at increased frequencies even at low-level muscle contractions. Another possible sign of re-innervation may come from polyphasic motor unit potentials, showing an increase in amplitude with a longer duration.

Our current study (Xu *et al.*, 2012) also shows that the LEMG characteristics of 35.6% patients with vocal fold immobility following endotracheal intubation are not completely normal. Nonetheless, the LEMG abnormality in 96.7% of patients was improved at the 1-month follow-up assessment after the reduction. Therefore, for patients with arytenoid dislocations from persistent and intractable nerve injuries and vocal fold paralysis.

## Diagnosis of myasthenia gravis using LEMG

Myasthenia gravis is caused by abnormal neuromuscular transmission at nerve junctions, resulting in clinical fatigable weaknesses in specific striated muscle groups. The diagnosis of myasthenia gravis requires the combination of clinical evaluation, pharmacological testing and electrophysiological study with EMG. Ocular weakness with asymmetric ptosis and binocular diplopia are typical initial presentations of myasthenia gravis. It has been noticed that some patients may have laryngeal problems as their initial symptoms of myasthenia gravis (Hartl et al., 2007; Liu et al., 2007; Mao et al., 2001). However, information on laryngeal nerve and related laryngeal muscle changes in the diagnosis of myasthenia gravis is scarce.

Our center conducted a prospective study that evaluated 32 subjects with myasthenia gravis. Laryngeal behaviors, voice assessment, characteristics of LEMG and repetitive nerve stimulation tests were carried out (Xu et al., 2009b). The repetitive nerve stimulation (RNS) test for the laryngeal muscle was performed using monopolar needle electrodes for stimulating the recurrent and superior laryngeal nerves at low frequencies (1 Hz, 3 Hz). All subjects demonstrated normal LEMG signals in conventional EMG. However, the amplitudes of the evoked LEMG were increased, especially in the TA and CT muscles. The durations of the evoked LEMG were nevertheless decreased significantly. The reason for this observation was not clear. We found that the RNS test for the laryngeal muscles had a high sensitivity (87.5%) in identifying myasthenia gravis (Xu et al., 2009b). The TA and CT muscles were more likely to demonstrate abnormal RNS findings than the other laryngeal muscles. Hence, we consider that combining the RNS test for TA and CT muscles with that for facial muscles or limb muscles can improve its sensitivity for the diagnosis of myasthenia gravis.

Undoubtedly, there are risks associated with the LEMG procedures. Laryngeal edema and/or bleeding are the most common complications. These problems may be alleviated by the use of hot packs and cold compression, corticosteroids or topical vasoconstrictors. In the cases of child subjects who require sedation or general anesthesia because of discomfort and fear of the use of needle placement (Jacobs & Finkel, 2002), the risks involved in the sedation or anesthetic should also be taken into consideration. The benefit of having a definitive diagnosis using LEMG for patients with suspected laryngeal neuromuscular disorders probably outweighs these risks.

## References

Amir, O., Ashkenazi, O., Leibovitzh, T., Michael, O., Tavor, Y. and Wolf, M. (2006) Applying the Voice Handicap Index (VHI) to dysphonic and nondysphonic Hebrew speakers. *Journal of Voice* 20 (2), 318–324.

Buchthal, F. (1959) Electromyography of intrinsic laryngeal muscles. *Journal of Experimental Physiology* 44, 137–148.

Deary, I.J., Wilson, J.A., Carding, P.N. and MacKenzie, K. (2003) VoiSS: A patient-derived voice symptom scale. *Journal of Psychosomatic Research* 54 (5), 483–489.

Duan, J., Zhu, L., Yan, Y., Pan, T., Lu, P. and Ma, F. (2010) The efficacy of a voice training program: A case-control study in China. *European Archives of Oto-Rhino-Laryngology* 267 (1), 101–105.

Faaborg-Andersen, K. and Buchthal, F. (1956) Action potentials from internal laryngeal muscles during phonation. *Nature* 177, 340–341.

Guimarães, I. and Abberton, E. (2004) An investigation of the Voice Handicap Index with speakers of Portuguese: Preliminary data. *Journal of Voice* 18 (1), 71–82.

Hakkesteegt, M.M., Wieringa, M.H., Gerritsma, E.J. and Feenstra, L. (2006) Reproducibility of the Dutch version of the Voice Handicap Index. *Folia Phoniatrica et Logopaedica* 58, 132–138.

Hartl, D.M., Leboulleux, S., Klap, P. and Schlumberger, M. (2007) Myasthenia gravis mimicking unilateral vocal fold paralysis at presentation. *Journal of Laryngology & Otology* 121, 174–178.

Hillel, A.D. (2001) The study of laryngeal muscle activity in normal human subjects and in patients with laryngeal dystonia using multiple fine-wire electromyography. *Laryngoscope* 111 (S97), 1–47.

Hirano, M. (1981) *Clinical Examination of Voice*. Vienna: Springer Verlag.

Hogikyan, N.D. and Sethuraman, G. (1999) Validation of an instrument to measure voice-related quality of life (V-RQOL). *Journal of Voice* 13 (4), 557–569.

Hsiung, M-W., Lu, P., Kang, B-H. and Wang, H-W. (2003) Measurement and validation of the Voice Handicap Index in voice-disordered patients in Taiwan. *Journal of Laryngology & Otology* 117, 478–481.

Jacobs, I.N. and Finkel, R.S. (2002) Laryngeal electromyography in the management of vocal cord mobility problems in children. *Laryngoscope* 112 (7), 1243–1248.

Jacobson, B.H., Johnson, A., Grywalski, C., Silbergleit, A., Jacobson, G., Benninger, M.S., et al. (1997) The Voice Handicap Index (VHI): Development and validation. *American Journal of Speech-Language Pathology* 6, 66–70.

Kimaid, P.A., Crespo, A.N., Quagliato, E.M., Wolf, A., Viana, M.A. and Resende, L.A. (2004) Laryngeal electromyography: Contribution to vocal fold immobility diagnosis. *Electromyography and Clinical Neurophysiology* 44 (6), 371–374.

Koufman, J.A., Postma, G.N., Whang, C.S., Rees, C.J., Amin, M.R., Belafsky, P.C., et al. (2001) Diagnostic laryngeal electromyography: The Wake Forest experience 1995–1999. *Otolaryngology – Head and Neck Surgery* 124 (6), 603–606.

Lam, P.K.Y., Chan, K.M., Ho, W.K., Kwong, E., Yiu, E.M. and Wei, W.I. (2006) Cross-cultural adaptation and validation of the Chinese Voice Handicap Index-10. *Laryngoscope* 116 (7), 1192–1198.

Li, H.Y., Xu, W., Han, D.M., Hu, R., Hu, H.Y., Hou, L.Z., et al. (2009) [Self-assessment characteristics of Voice Handicap Index for voice disorders and its influencing factors]. *Zhonghua Er Bi Yan Hou Tou Jing Wai Ke Za Zhi* 44 (2), 109–113 [in Chinese].

Li, H., Huang, Z., Hu, R., Zhang, L. and Xu, W. (2012) Study on the simplified Chinese version of the Voice Handicap Index. *Journal of Voice* 26 (3), 365–371.

Liu, W-B., Xia, Q., Men, L-N., Wu, Z-K. and Huang, R-X. (2007) Dysphonia as a primary manifestation in myasthenia gravis (MG): A retrospective review of 7 cases among 1520 MG patients. *Journal of the Neurological Sciences* 260 (1–2), 16–22.

Mao, V.H., Abaza, M. and Spiegel, J.R. (2001) Laryngeal myasthenia gravis: Report of 40 cases. *Journal of Voice* 15 (1), 122–130.

Mu, L. and Yang, S. (1991) An experimental study on the laryngeal electromyography and visual observations in varying types of surgical injuries to the unilateral recurrent laryngeal nerve in the neck. *Laryngoscope* 101 (7), 699–708.

Rosen, C.A., Lee, A.S., Osborne, J., Zullo, T. and Murry, T. (2004) Development and validation of the Voice Handicap Index-10. *Laryngoscope* 114 (9), 1549–1556.

Sataloff, R.T., Mandel, S., Mann, E.A. and Ludlow, C.L. (2004) Practice parameter: Laryngeal electromyography (an evidence-based review). *Otolaryngology – Head and Neck Surgery* 130 (6), 770–779.

Sataloff, R.T., Praneetvatakul, P., Heuer, R.J., Hawkshaw, M.J., Heman-Ackah, Y.D., Schneider, S.M., *et al.* (2010) Laryngeal electromyography: Clinical application. *Journal of Voice* 24 (2), 228–234.

Wang, L.M., Zhu, Q., Ma, T., Li, J.P., Hu, R., Rong, X.Y., *et al.* (2011) Value of ultrasonography in diagnosis of pediatric vocal fold paralysis. *International Journal of Pediatric Otorhinolaryngology* 75 (9), 1186–1190.

Xu, W., Han, D., Hou, L., Zhang, L. and Zhao, G. (2007) Value of laryngeal electromyography in diagnosis of vocal fold immobility. *Annals of Otology, Rhinology, and Laryngology* 116 (8), 576–581.

Xu, W., Li, H.Y., Hu, R., Hu, H.Y., Hou, L.Z., Zhang, L., *et al.* (2008) [Analysis of reliability and validity of the Chinese version of Voice Handicap Index (VHI)]. *Zhonghua Er Bi Yan Hou Tou Jing Wai Ke Za Zhi* 43 (9), 670–675 [in Chinese].

Xu, W., Han, D., Hu, H., Chen, X., Li, H., Hou, L., *et al.* (2009a) Endoscopic mucosal suturing of vocal fold with placement of stent for the treatment of glottic stenoses. *Head & Neck* 31 (6), 732–737.

Xu, W., Han, D., Hou, L., Hu, R. and Wang, L. (2009b) Clinical and electrophysiological characteristics of larynx in myasthenia gravis. *Annals of Otology, Rhinology, and Laryngology* 118 (9), 656–661.

Xu, W., Han, D., Li, H., Hu, R. and Zhang, L. (2010) Application of the Mandarin Chinese version of the Voice Handicap Index. *Journal of Voice* 24 (6), 702–707.

Xu, W., Han, D., Hu, R., Bai, Y. and Zhang, L. (2012) Characteristics of vocal fold immobility following endotracheal intubation. *Annals of Otology, Rhinology, and Laryngology.*

Yin, S.S., Qiu, W.W. and Stucker, F.J. (1997) Major patterns of laryngeal electromyography and their clinical application. *Laryngoscope* 107 (1), 126–136.

# Appendix 4.1 Mandarin Chinese Version of the VHI and its Translation into English (Xu *et al.*, 2010)

## 嗓 音 障 碍 指 数 量 表
### VOICE HANDICAP INDEX (VHI)

为评估发声问题对您生活的影响程度，请在认为符合自己情况的数字上划圈：

| 0=无； | 1=很少； | 2=有时； | 3=经常； | 4=总是 |

**第一部分　功能方面（FUNCTIONAL）：**

| | | | | | | |
|---|---|---|---|---|---|---|
| F1 | 由于我的嗓音问题别人难以听见我说话的声音 | 0 | 1 | 2 | 3 | 4 |
| F2 | 在嘈杂环境中别人难以听明白我说的话 | 0 | 1 | 2 | 3 | 4 |
| F3 | 当我在房间另一头叫家人时，他们难以听见 | 0 | 1 | 2 | 3 | 4 |
| F7 | 面对面交谈时，别人会要我重复我说过的话 | 0 | 1 | 2 | 3 | 4 |

由于噪音问题：

| | | | | | | |
|---|---|---|---|---|---|---|
| F4 | 我打电话的次数较以往减少 | 0 | 1 | 2 | 3 | 4 |
| F5 | 我会刻意避免在人多的地方与人交谈 | 0 | 1 | 2 | 3 | 4 |
| F6 | 我减少与朋友、邻居或亲人说话 | 0 | 1 | 2 | 3 | 4 |
| F8 | 限制了我的个人及社交生活 | 0 | 1 | 2 | 3 | 4 |
| F9 | 我感到在交谈中话跟不上 | 0 | 1 | 2 | 3 | 4 |
| F10 | 我的收入受到影响 | 0 | 1 | 2 | 3 | 4 |

**第二部分　生理方面（PHYSICAL）：**

| | | | | | | |
|---|---|---|---|---|---|---|
| P1 | 说话时我会感觉气短 | 0 | 1 | 2 | 3 | 4 |
| P2 | 一天之中我的嗓音不稳定，会有变化 | 0 | 1 | 2 | 3 | 4 |
| P3 | 人们会问我："你的声音出了什么问题？" | 0 | 1 | 2 | 3 | 4 |
| P4 | 我的声音听上去嘶哑干涩 | 0 | 1 | 2 | 3 | 4 |
| P5 | 我感到好像需要努力才能发出声音 | 0 | 1 | 2 | 3 | 4 |
| P6 | 我声音的清晰度变化无常 | 0 | 1 | 2 | 3 | 4 |
| P7 | 我会尝试改变我的声音以便听起来有所不同 | 0 | 1 | 2 | 3 | 4 |
| P8 | 我说话时感到很吃力 | 0 | 1 | 2 | 3 | 4 |
| P9 | 我的声音晚上会更差 | 0 | 1 | 2 | 3 | 4 |
| P10 | 我说话时会出现失声的情况 | 0 | 1 | 2 | 3 | 4 |

**第三部分　情感方面（EMOTIONAL）：**

| | | | | | | |
|---|---|---|---|---|---|---|
| E1 | 我的声音使我在与他人交谈时感到紧张 | 0 | 1 | 2 | 3 | 4 |
| E2 | 别人听到我的声音会觉得难受 | 0 | 1 | 2 | 3 | 4 |
| E3 | 我发现别人并不能理解我的声音问题 | 0 | 1 | 2 | 3 | 4 |

由于噪音问题：

| | | | | | | |
|---|---|---|---|---|---|---|
| E4 | 我感到苦恼 | 0 | 1 | 2 | 3 | 4 |
| E5 | 我变得不如以前外向 | 0 | 1 | 2 | 3 | 4 |
| E6 | 我觉得自己身体有缺陷 | 0 | 1 | 2 | 3 | 4 |
| E7 | 别人让我重复刚说过的话时，我感到烦恼 | 0 | 1 | 2 | 3 | 4 |
| E8 | 别人让我重复刚说过的话时，我感到尴尬 | 0 | 1 | 2 | 3 | 4 |
| E9 | 觉得自己能力不够（没有用） | 0 | 1 | 2 | 3 | 4 |
| E10 | 我感到羞愧 | 0 | 1 | 2 | 3 | 4 |

# Translation of the Chinese version of the VHI into English

## voice handicap index

*Instructions*: In order to describe the degree to which the problem with your voice has affected your life, please circle the numbers that you feel apply most closely.

0 = Never   1 = Seldom   2 = Sometimes   3 = Almost always   4 = Always

### Part 1. Functional

| | | |
|---|---|---|
| F1: | It is difficult for others to hear me because of my voice. | 0 1 2 3 4 |
| F2: | It is difficult for others to understand me in a noisy room. | 0 1 2 3 4 |
| F3: | My family has difficulty hearing me when I call them in the other room. | 0 1 2 3 4 |
| F7: | People ask me to repeat when talking face to face. | 0 1 2 3 4 |

Because of my voice:

| | | |
|---|---|---|
| F4: | I use the telephone less often. | 0 1 2 3 4 |
| F5: | I tend to avoid talking with many people. | 0 1 2 3 4 |
| F6: | I talk with my friends, neighbors and relatives less than before. | 0 1 2 3 4 |
| F8: | My voice restricts my personal and social life. | 0 1 2 3 4 |
| F9: | I feel it's difficult for me to join in a conversation. | 0 1 2 3 4 |
| F10: | I get less income. | 0 1 2 3 4 |

### Part 2. Physical

| | | |
|---|---|---|
| P1: | I feel I run out of air when I talk. | 0 1 2 3 4 |
| P2: | The sound of my voice varies during a day. | 0 1 2 3 4 |
| P3: | People ask me: 'What's wrong with your voice?' | 0 1 2 3 4 |
| P4: | My voice sounds dry and hoarse. | 0 1 2 3 4 |
| P5: | I feel I must push to produce my voice. | 0 1 2 3 4 |
| P6: | The clarity of my voice is unstable. | 0 1 2 3 4 |
| P7: | I try to change my voice to make it sound different (better). | 0 1 2 3 4 |
| P8: | It takes me a lot of effort to speak. | 0 1 2 3 4 |
| P9: | My voice is worse in the evening. | 0 1 2 3 4 |
| P10: | My voice goes away in the middle of speaking. | 0 1 2 3 4 |

### Part 3. Emotional

| | | |
|---|---|---|
| E1: | I am nervous when I talk with others because of my voice. | 0 1 2 3 4 |
| E2: | People feel unhappy because of my voice. | 0 1 2 3 4 |
| E3: | I find others can't understand why my voice is like that. | 0 1 2 3 4 |

Because of my voice:

| | | |
|---|---|---|
| E4: | It upsets me. | 0  1  2  3  4 |
| E5: | I am less extroverted than before. | 0  1  2  3  4 |
| E6: | I feel handicapped. | 0  1  2  3  4 |
| E7: | I feel annoyed when people ask me to repeat. | 0  1  2  3  4 |
| E8: | I feel embarrassed when people ask me to repeat. | 0  1  2  3  4 |
| E9: | I feel incompetent (useless). | 0  1  2  3  4 |
| E10: | I feel ashamed. | 0  1  2  3  4 |

# Appendix 4.2 The Items of the Simplified Chinese Version VHI-7, VHI-10 and VHI-13

*Instructions*: Please circle the numbers that best describe the impact of the voice disorder on your life.

0 = Never   1 = Seldom   2 = Sometimes   3 = Almost always   4 = Always

*VHI-7*

| | | |
|---|---|---|
| F2: | It is difficult for others to understand me in a noisy room. | 0  1  2  3  4 |
| F9: | I feel it is difficult for me to join a conversation. | 0  1  2  3  4 |
| P9: | I feel I run out of air when I talk. | 0  1  2  3  4 |
| P2: | The sound of my voice varies during a day. | 0  1  2  3  4 |
| P3: | People ask me: 'What's wrong with your voice?' | 0  1  2  3  4 |
| P6: | The clarity of my voice is unstable. | 0  1  2  3  4 |
| E4: | It upsets me. | 0  1  2  3  4 |

*The additional items of VHI-10*

| | | |
|---|---|---|
| F6: | I talk with my friends, neighbors and relatives less than before. | 0  1  2  3  4 |
| P10: | My voice goes away in the middle of speaking. | 0  1  2  3  4 |
| E2: | People feel unhappy because of my voice. | 0  1  2  3  4 |

*The additional items of VHI-13*

| | | |
|---|---|---|
| P7: | I try to change my voice to make it sound different (better). | 0  1  2  3  4 |
| P9: | My voice is worse in the evening. | 0  1  2  3  4 |
| E5: | I am less extroverted than before. | 0  1  2  3  4 |

# 5 Current Issues in Voice Assessment and Intervention in Hong Kong

Estella P-M. Ma and Triska K-Y. Lee

## Introduction

Before 1980 there was no speech therapy/pathology training course in Hong Kong. All the qualified speech therapists in Hong Kong received their professional training overseas from Australia, North America and the United Kingdom. Voice assessment and treatment in Hong Kong have been strongly influenced by the models and practices developed in western countries. However, the differences in language and culture between Hong Kong and the western countries have introduced challenges when adopting these western models to a Hong Kong context. This chapter will first give an overview of voice problems and the healthcare system in Hong Kong. It will then discuss current issues of voice assessment and treatment within the context of Hong Kong. The final section of the chapter will look ahead to the setting out of a research agenda for the future development of voice assessment and treatment in Hong Kong.

## Overview of Voice Problems in Hong Kong

Hong Kong is a highly urbanised city with a population of over seven million at the end of 2010 (HKSAR Census and Statistics Department, 2011). Voice problems are common in Hong Kong. The majority of voice disorders are related to phonotrauma due to the overuse or misuse of the voice. Several studies have reported the prevalence data of voice problems among teachers in Hong Kong. An early study conducted in Hong Kong recorded clinical caseload data on 115 treatment-seeking patients in public speech therapy clinics. Teachers comprised around one-fifth of the voice caseload (Yiu & Ho, 1991). A small-scale longitudinal study followed 52 high school teacher trainees for five years after graduation. One-third of the teachers who had been teaching for two years experienced voice problems, and 21% of them reported that they had taken more than three days off work annually because of their voice problems (Chan *et al.*, 2005). Another survey conducted by Chung and Chan (2007) revealed a much higher percentage (73.5%) of teachers with voice problems. These prevalence figures of voice problems in teachers are comparable to those reported in western countries such as the UK and the USA.

## Overview of the Healthcare System in Hong Kong

Hong Kong used to be a British colony and was governed by the British government before its reversion to Chinese sovereignty in July 1997. From July 1997 Hong Kong became a special administrative region of China. Nevertheless, Hong Kong inherited the public-funded healthcare system of the former British government. Under the current healthcare system in Hong Kong, the public healthcare service is primarily delivered by public hospitals. Patients with voice problems are seen under the allied health services provided by Specialist Outpatient Clinics (SOPC) of the hospital. This sector is usually affiliated to either the ear, nose and throat (oto-rhino-laryngology) or the speech therapy department. The consultation fee is highly subsidised, with a current initial consultation fee of HK$100 (approximately US$12.5) and subsequent attendance fees of HK$60 (approximately US$7.5) in specialist outpatient clinics. Due to the highly subsidised healthcare system, the demand for voice therapy in the public sector is very high, as is indicated by the long waiting list for the service. In major public hospitals it is not uncommon to wait at least six months to receive voice therapy for hyperfunctional voice-disordered cases. Therefore many voice patients turn to private voice clinics. Consultation fees in private voice clinics are generally much higher than in public hospitals and can vary across clinics. Children with voice problems who are studying in mainstream primary schools receive speech therapy services through the school-based support programmes offered by the Hong Kong government.

In Hong Kong, a professional involved in speech pathology practice is called a speech therapist. This terminology is slightly different from that used in other countries such as Australia (speech pathologist), the UK (speech and language therapist) and the USA (speech-language pathologist). Speech therapists practising in Hong Kong abide by the Code of Ethics and Standard of Practice which guide the clinical practice of the Hong Kong Association of Speech Therapists (HKAST; http://www.speechtherapy.org.hk). As of 2012 there are approximately 650 practising speech therapists in Hong Kong.

# Issues Related to Voice Assessment in Hong Kong

In Hong Kong, clinical routine assessment of voice-disordered clients follows the general practice in the USA (see the chapter in this book by Eadie and Hapner). Every voice client is supposed to be evaluated by both an otolaryngologist and a speech therapist. The otolaryngologist performs functional and structural evaluation of the client's laryngeal and peri-laryngeal structures. The evaluation is usually done indirectly, either by laryngeal mirror or videoendoscopy. Videostroboscopy may be used for a more detailed examination of vocal fold functions and structures during phonation. The speech therapist performs a clinical history interview with the client to explore the client's voice use patterns, any contributing factors and the nature of the voice problems. The severity of the voice problems is then assessed by auditory-perceptual evaluation and often by instrumental measurements.

In recent years there has been increased attention on the impacts of voice impairment on one's quality of life within the clinical management of voice disorders. The World Health Organization health classification scheme – International Classification of Functioning, Disability and Health (ICF; WHO, 2001) – has been adopted by the speech therapy/pathology profession as an overarching framework for the management of communication disorders (see Ma et al., 2007a; Worrall et al., 2008 for details). This framework describes the consequences of a disorder in terms of impairment, activity limitation and participation restriction. The framework also emphasises the roles of contextual factors (environmental and personal) in influencing the functioning and disability of the individual. Ma and colleagues (2007b) have discussed how the ICF can be applied to the assessment and treatment of voice disorders. The framework promotes a holistic approach when working with individuals with voice problems by extending the traditional focus on vocal fold structures and functions to an additional consideration of the functional impacts due to voice problems.

One key issue of clinical voice assessment in Hong Kong relates to the linguistic features of its major spoken language. In Hong Kong, Cantonese is the major spoken language. It is a dialect of Chinese and is a tone language. In a tone language, the pitch patterns (lexical tones) determine the lexical meaning of the syllable. For example, there are six contrastive tones in Cantonese. The syllable /ma/ means 'mother' when produced with a high steady pitch (high-level tone or tone 1) but means 'horse' when produced with a falling-then-rising pitch (low-rising tone or tone 5). On the contrary, most western European languages such as English are non-tone languages. The literature has documented that voice measures can manifest differently between tone and non-tone languages. For example, a greater fundamental frequency speaking range has been reported in American English speakers when compared to speakers of tone languages like Mandarin Chinese (Chen, 1972, 2005) and

Japanese (Yamazawa & Hollien, 1992). In terms of auditory-perceptual voice evaluation, the major language spoken by the listener may affect his/her perception of voice quality parameters and severity (Anders *et al.*, 1988).

The above-mentioned linguistic features of Cantonese pose two implications for voice assessment in Hong Kong. Firstly, the normative data reported in the literature in the early years, gathered from western populations with English-speaking individuals, are not applicable to the Cantonese population. Secondly, there is a need to develop a language-specific evaluation tool for the Cantonese-speaking population. In order to deal with these issues, a number of voice assessment tools have been developed and validated. These tools have greatly facilitated the establishment of normative data for the Hong Kong Cantonese population.

## Voice Activity and Participation Profile

The Voice Activity and Participation Profile (VAPP; Ma & Yiu, 2001) was developed around the conceptual framework of the International Classification of Impairments, Activities and Participation (ICIDH-2 Beta-1; WHO, 1997), which preceded the ICF. The VAPP is a 28-item self-assessing questionnaire ascertaining the extents of functional limitations and restrictions in carrying out voice activities because of voice problems. The impacts are evaluated in four domains: effects on jobs, daily communication, social communication and emotion. The VAPP has been demonstrated to be a sensitive tool in identifying possible differences in perception of voice-related functional impacts in individuals from different cultures (Yiu *et al.*, 2011).

## Training programme for auditory-perceptual voice evaluation

This training programme (Chan & Yiu, 2002; Yiu *et al.*, 2007a) uses synthesised voice stimuli as external voice anchors to improve rating reliability between listeners. The synthesised voice stimuli were based on a prototype sentence in Cantonese which covers normal, mild, moderate and severe levels of breathiness and roughness qualities. The programme uses a stimulus-response-stimulus-feedback training paradigm.

## Cantonese version of the Voice Handicap Index

The Voice Handicap Index (VHI) was originally developed in English by Jacobson and colleagues (1997). The impacts of voice disorders are assessed in terms of functional, physical and emotional areas. During the validation process of the Cantonese version of the VHI, Lam *et al.* (2006) reported differences in scores between those obtained in Hong Kong and those reported by Rosen *et al.* (2004). These differences in scores might have been contributed to by the cultural and environmental differences between Hong Kong and western countries.

## Normative data for aerodynamic and acoustic voice measures

A number of studies using normative data for Cantonese speakers have been reported. Readers can refer to the individual reports for details of the normative data: Ma and Yiu (2005, 2006); Ma et al. (2007c, in press); Yiu et al. (2004).

# Issues Related to Voice Treatment in Hong Kong

The majority of the voice caseloads in Hong Kong are related to hyperfunctional voice disorders. Conservative voice therapy is considered as the first line of treatment for patients with laryngeal pathologies associated with hyperfunctional voice use (Yiu et al., 2007b). Phonosurgery may be recommended for more severe cases or as a last resort for recalcitrant cases. A conservative voice therapy programme usually runs for between six and eight sessions, covering both indirect and direct voice therapy. The programme begins with vocal hygiene education, which focuses on eliminating vocal behaviours that are believed to contribute to the voice problem. A local, unpublished survey reported that vocal hygiene education is the most commonly used therapeutic technique among speech therapists in Hong Kong (Lo, 2000). Apart from vocal hygiene education, various vocal facilitative techniques are used to facilitate effective phonation, with the goal of minimising the risks of phonotrauma and hence optimising wound healing. Humming, a variant of resonant voice therapy, is a frequently used technique in voice clinics in Hong Kong (Yiu, 2008). The decision to use individual versus group therapy depends on the caseload of the clinics and it varies across clinical settings.

Geographically, Hong Kong is located on the southern part of mainland China. Although Hong Kong has a long history of development in western medicine, it has also been influenced by the concept of traditional Chinese medicine. For example, alternative and complementary medicine has been adopted for treating voice problems associated with benign vocal pathologies. At the Voice Research Laboratory, randomised controlled trials have been carried out to evaluate the effects of acupuncture in treating vocal pathologies related to phonotrauma. The findings showed that acupuncture at the appropriate acupoints is effective in treating benign vocal fold lesions, including vocal nodules and polyps (Kwong & Yiu, 2010; Yiu et al., 2006).

# Future Development of Voice Assessment and Treatment Research in Hong Kong

This section will discuss three areas for future development in voice assessment and treatment research that are relevant to the Hong Kong context. These areas are: (1) expanding normative voice data for various age groups; (2) implementing preventive work for voice problems; and (3) implementing alternative service delivery models of voice therapy.

## Expanding normative voice data for various age groups

There are significant differences between the laryngeal structures of adults, children and the elderly. Therefore, normative data developed within the adult population cannot be applied to children and the elderly. Unfortunately, both children and the elderly population are currently under-researched. A comprehensive normative database of the Cantonese-speaking population, particularly focusing on both the paediatric and geriatric populations, would be useful for the assessment of voice problems in these populations.

## Implementing preventive work for voice problems

Educational voice programmes which promote healthy voice use habits have been shown to be effective in preventing voice problems among high-risk groups such as schoolteachers (Chan, 1994; Morton & Watson, 1998) and young children (Aaron & Madison, 1991; Nilson & Schneiderman, 1983). Some universities and institutes in Singapore and the UK have already included voice protection programmes as compulsory training courses for student teachers. Currently in Hong Kong there is no systematic mechanism to equip schoolteachers with voice care knowledge during their course of training or career. Similarly, for young children, voice care education is not integrated in the school curriculum in Hong Kong. There is a need for more preventative work for voice problems.

## Implementing alternative service delivery models of voice therapy

Traditionally, voice therapy is provided on a face-to-face basis. Unlike countries with rural areas, Hong Kong is a highly urbanised region, so physical accessibility to the clinical service is not an issue. Nevertheless, many clients attending our clinics reported that their busy lifestyle and heavy job duties lowered their motivation for and adherence to attendance at voice therapy sessions. It is therefore not surprising to see a low treatment-seeking rate, despite the high prevalence rates of voice problems. Advances in telecommunication technology can facilitate the application of telehealth rehabilitation in the management of voice-disordered cases. The use of telehealth in delivering voice therapy allows greater flexibility in time and venue. Telehealth has been increasingly used as a means of service delivery of speech and voice therapy. There have been several telehealth applications developed to assess and treat individuals with communication disorders, including motor speech disorders in individuals with Parkinson's disease (Theodoros *et al.*, 2006), voice problems in adults (Mashima *et al.*, 2003) and swallowing functions in laryngectomies (Ward *et al.*, 2007). The use of home-based multimedia packages for treating teachers with voice problems has also been demonstrated to be effective (Chan, 2008).

# Conclusions

In summary, this chapter presents an overview of the voice problems and health care system in Hong Kong. Several issues related to the clinical assessment and treatment of voice problems within a Hong Kong setting are discussed. Currently, a series of research projects is being carried out at the Voice Research Laboratory at the University of Hong Kong (such as preventive voice programmes for teachers, the application of a telehealth approach in providing voice therapy, and the application of traditional Chinese medicine in treating voice problems). It is hopeful that such translational research will contribute to the empirical evidence for clinical best practice, with the ultimate goal of improving the quality of life in individuals with voice problems.

## References

Aaron, V.L. and Madison, C.L. (1991) A vocal hygiene program for high-school cheerleaders. *Language, Speech, and Hearing Services in Schools* 22, 287–290.

Anders, L.C., Hollien, H., Hurme, P., Sonninen, A. and Wendler, J. (1988) Perception of hoarseness by several classes of listeners. *Folia Phoniatrica et Logopaedica* 40, 91–100.

Chan, K.M-K. and Yiu, E.M-L. (2002) The effect of anchors and training on the reliability of perceptual voice evaluation. *Journal of Speech, Language and Hearing Research* 45 (1), 111–126.

Chan, K., Yiu, E. and Ma, E. (2005) A longitudinal study on the occurrence and impact of voice problems on teachers. Paper presented at the Voice Foundation's 34th Annual Symposium, Philadelphia.

Chan, M.S-K. (2008) Effectiveness of a multimedia-based voice therapy program for teachers with voice disorders. Unpublished MPhil thesis, University of Hong Kong.

Chan, R.W.K. (1994) Does the voice improve with vocal hygiene education? A study of some instrumental voice measures in a group of kindergarten teachers. *Journal of Voice* 8 (3), 279–291.

Chen, G.T. (1972) A comparative study of pitch range of native speakers of Midwestern English and Mandarin Chinese: An acoustic study. Doctoral dissertation, University of Wisconsin-Madison.

Chen, S.H. (2005) The effects of tones on speaking frequency and intensity ranges in Mandarin and Min dialects. *Journal of Acoustical Society of America* 117, 3225–3230.

Chung, Y.L. and Chan, H.T. (2007) Occupational health problems in Hong Kong primary and secondary school teachers. Hong Kong Occupational Safety & Health Bureau, *Green Cross* January/February.

HKSAR Census and Statistics Department (2011) Hong Kong statistics. Online at http://www.censtatd.gov.hk/hong_kong_statistics/statistics_by_subject/index.jsp?subjectID=1&charsetID=1&displayMode=T#FOOTNOTE1

Jacobson, B.H., Johnson, A., Grywalski, C., Silbergleit, A., Jacobson, G., Benninger, M.S., et al. (1997) The Voice Handicap Index (VHI): Development and validation. *American Journal of Speech-Language Pathology* 6 (3), 66–70.

Kwong, E.Y.-L. and Yiu, E.M-L. (2010) A preliminary study of the effect of acupuncture on salivary cortisol level in female dysphonic speakers. *Journal of Voice* 24 (6), 719–723.

Lam, P.K.Y., Chan, K.M., Ho, W., Kwong, E., Yiu, E.M. and Wei, W.I. (2006) Cross-cultural adaptation and validation of the Chinese Voice Handicap Index-10. *Laryngoscope* 116, 1192–1198.

Lo, C.O-Y. (2000) Differences in management strategies for hyperfunctional voice disorders between speech therapists and student speech therapists. Unpublished BSc dissertation, University of Hong Kong.

Ma, E.P-M. and Yiu, E.M-L. (2001) Voice activity and participation profile: Assessing the impact of voice disorders on daily activities. *Journal of Speech, Language and Hearing Research* 44 (3), 511–524.

Ma, E.P-M. and Yiu, E.M-L. (2005) Suitability of acoustic perturbation measures in analyzing periodic and nearly periodic voice signals. *Folia Phoniatrica et Logopaedica* 57 (1), 38–47.

Ma, E.P-M. and Yiu, E.M-L. (2006) Multi-parametric evaluation of dysphonic severity. *Journal of Voice* 20 (3), 380–390.

Ma, E.P-M., Worrall, L. and Threats, T.T. (2007a) The International Classification of Functioning, Disability and Health (ICF) in clinical practice. *Seminars in Speech and Language* 28 (4), 241–243.

Ma, E.P-M., Yiu, E.M-L. and Verdolini Abbott, K. (2007b) Application of the ICF in voice disorders. *Seminars in Speech and Language* 28 (4), 343–350.

Ma, E., Robertson, J., Radford, C., Vagne, S., El-Halabi, R. and Yiu, E. (2007c) Reliability of speaking and maximum voice range measures in screening for dysphonia. *Journal of Voice* 21 (4), 397–406.

Ma, E.P-M., Baken, R.J., Roark, R.M. and Li, P-M. (in press) Effect of tones on vocal attack time (VAT) in Cantonese speakers. *Journal of Voice*.

Mashima, P.A., Birkmire-Peters, D.P., Syms, M.J., Holtel, M.R., Burgess, L.P.A. and Peters, L.J. (2003) Telehealth: Voice therapy using telecommunications technology. *American Journal of Speech-Language Pathology* 12, 432–439.

Morton, V. and Watson, D.R. (1998) The teaching voice: Problems and perceptions. *Logopedics Phoniatrics Vocology* 23, 133–139.

Nilson, H. and Schneiderman, C.R. (1983) Classroom program for the prevention of vocal abuse and hoarseness in elementary school children. *Language, Speech, and Hearing Services in Schools* 14 (2), 121–127.

Rosen, C.A., Lee, A.S., Osborne, J., Zullo, T. and Murry, T. (2004) Development and validation of the Voice Handicap Index-10. *Laryngoscope* 114, 1549–1556.

Theodoros, D.G., Constantinescu, G., Russell, T.G., Ward, E.C., Wilson, S.J. and Wootton, R. (2006) Treating the speech disorder in Parkinson's disease online. *Journal of Telemedicine and Telecare* 12 (3), 88–91.

Ward, L., White, J., Russell, T., Theodoros, D., Kuhl, M., Nelson, K., et al. (2007) Assessment of communication and swallowing function post laryngectomy: A telerehabilitation trial. *Journal of Telemedicine and Telecare* 13 (3), 88–91.

Worrall, L.E., Ma, E.P-M. and Threats, T.T. (2008) Contribution of the ICF to speech-language pathology. *International Journal of Speech-Language Pathology,* 10 (1–2).

Yamazawa, H. and Hollien, H. (1992) Speaking fundamental frequency patterns of Japanese women. *Phonetica* 49, 128–140.

Yiu, E. (2008) Hong Kong humming. In A. Behrman and J. Haskell (eds) *Exercises for Voice Therapy* (pp. 85–86). San Diego: Plural Publishing.

Yiu, E.M-L. and Ho, P.S-P. (1991) Voice problems in Hong Kong: A preliminary report. *Australian Journal of Human Communication Disorders* 19, 45–58.

Yiu, E.M-L., Yuen, Y-M., Whitehill, T. and Winkworth, A. (2004) Reliability and applicability of aerodynamic measures in dysphonia assessment. *Clinical Linguistics and Phonetics* 18 (6–8), 463–478.

Yiu, E., Xu, J.J., Murry, T., Wei, W.I., Yu, M., Ma, E., *et al.* (2006) A randomized treatment-placebo study of the effectiveness of acupuncture for benign vocal pathologies. *Journal of Voice* 20 (1), 144–156.

Yiu, E.M-L., Chan, K.M-K. and Mok, R.S-M. (2007a) Reliability and confidence in using a paired comparison paradigm in perceptual voice quality evaluation. *Clinical Linguistics & Phonetics* 21 (2), 129–145.

Yiu, E.M-L., Wei, W., van Hasselt, A. and Wong, R. (2007b) Predicting the outcome of conservative (non-surgical) voice therapy for adults with laryngeal pathologies associated with hyperfunctional voice use. *Hong Kong Medical Journal* 13 (5, Suppl. 5), 15–17.

Yiu, E.M. L., Ho, E.M., Ma, E.P.M., Verdolini Abbott, K., Branski, R., Richardson, K., *et al.* (2011) Possible cross-cultural differences in the perception of impact of voice disorders. *Journal of Voice* 25 (3), 348–353.

WHO (1997) *International Classification of Impairments, Activities, and Participation. A Manual of Dimensions of Disablement and Functioning. ICIDH-2, Beta-1 Draft for Field Trials.* Geneva: World Health Organization.

WHO (2001) *International Classification of Functioning, Disability and Health (ICF).* Geneva: World Health Organization.

# 6 Current Issues in Voice Assessment and Intervention in Israel

## Ofer Amir

The prevalence of voice disorders in Israel has never been evaluated systematically. The prevalence data on voice disorders in the general population range between 0.65% (Morley, 1952) to 15% (Laguaite, 1972). In a recent local survey conducted in Israel it was reported that 15.8% of 610 naïve respondents in the age range of 20–70 years felt they had a voice problem. One-third of them (34%) reported having hoarseness over the past year (Amir, 2011). These findings show that the prevalence of voice disorders in Israel is similar to that observed in other western developed countries.

It appears that the overall awareness of voice disorders, their impact on the quality of life and possibilities for treatment is relatively low in Israel. 'World Voice Day' was only recently recognised in Israel for the first time in 2010. The relatively low awareness of voice disorders, their possible impact on the quality of life and available treatment possibilities leads to low rates of dysphonic individuals seeking help and thus delays diagnosis and treatment. This chapter will first describe the voice therapy profession within the medical system in Israel. This will be followed by a discussion on the standards for laryngeal examination and voice therapy in Israel. This chapter will conclude with a discussion of the future of the voice profession in Israel.

The standard evaluation of voice disorders in Israel, similarly to other countries, includes a medical and laryngeal examination performed by an otolaryngologist and a functional voice evaluation performed by a speech pathologist. The Israeli medical system does not grant a sub-specialty of laryngology within the field of otorhinolaryngology. Therefore, all certified ear, nose and throat (ENT) physicians are allowed to perform a laryngeal examination. Over recent years, a growing yet small number of Israeli ENT physicians have developed advanced expertise in laryngology, following periods of fellowship in professional centres in various European countries or in the USA. Similarly, the Israeli medical system certifies speech pathologists to perform functional voice evaluations and subsequent voice therapy.

Nonetheless, this does not provide the grounds for defining a sub-specialty of voice therapy within the field of speech-language therapy or communication disorders. Hence, all speech-pathologists are allowed to perform functional voice evaluations and therapy.

Speech-pathology, in Israel, is considered to be one facet of the communication disorders profession. As such, graduates of an Israeli academic program of Communication Disorders are certified (following a national certification exam conducted by the Ministry of Health) in speech and language pathology and therapy, as well as in audiology. The academic studies, a three-and-a-half year program, are conducted at three recognised academic institutions (two universities and one college), while two other institutions are striving for academic accreditation. This program includes a single course (two semesters) on voice disorders and voice therapy, and a short (8 hours) practice of basic voice production and voice therapy techniques. Fulfilling these requirements entitles the graduates of these programs to perform voice evaluation and conduct voice therapy. Consequently, many voice clinicians feel a lack of clinical and theoretical knowledge when confronting complex cases or clients with psychogenic voice disorders. It should be noted that only recently was a state law approved, after a long process of nearly 20 years, which defines voice disorders as one of the professional fields within the responsibility of speech pathologists (defined in Israel as communication disorders clinicians).

## Laryngeal Examination in Israel

In Israel, laryngeal examination can only be performed by an ENT physician. Most dysphonic patients would firstly consult with a general practitioner or their family doctor, who would then refer them to an ENT physician, after an initial evaluation. The Israeli public healthcare system covers both exams, so there is no cost to the client for this examination. Nevertheless, the appointment time for an initial evaluation usually takes up to three months.

The majority of ENT physicians still perform indirect laryngoscopy using a mirror. Over the past decade, laryngoscopy with flexible or rigid laryngoscopes has become more common. This is more usual in private settings and in large medical centres that specialise in voice disorders. To date, high-speed laryngoscopy or video-kymography is not yet available as a routine procedure. After the ENT examination, appropriate referral is made. Options would include voice therapy, medical therapy, surgery or a combination of these.

## Voice Evaluation in Israel

In Israel, functional and perceptual evaluation of voice disorders is considered to fall within the responsibility and professional knowledge of speech pathologists. Prior to the initial referral to the speech pathologist, the client is expected to undergo a laryngeal examination by an ENT physician, and preferably to have a stroboscopic examination done by an ENT physician who specialises in laryngology. In clinical settings, the voice evaluation is performed by the speech pathologist, at his or her office, independently of the ENT physician's laryngeal examination. Although the clinical advantage of a concurrent voice evaluation by a laryngologist and a speech pathologist is acknowledged by most professionals in Israel, there is currently only one medical centre in Israel which adopts this as a routine practice in the voice clinic.

The Israeli medical system does not acknowledge a sub-specialty in voice within the field of speech pathology or communication disorders. Therefore, all certified speech pathologists in Israel are allowed to perform voice therapy. In practice, only a small number of them actively perform voice therapy. This can be reflected in some informal observations. For example, of the 900 speech pathologists and audiologists who attended the 2011 National Conference of the Israeli Speech, Language and Hearing Association (ISHLA; http://www.ishla.org.il), only 60 attended the voice session. In addition, of the 150 proposals submitted for presentations at the conference, only six were directly related to voice or voice therapy. Another observation from the Israeli Speech and Hearing Association online private practitioners' lists reveals on its website that only 64 out of a total of 360 speech pathologists regard themselves as practicing voice therapy among other speech pathology areas. Clearly, voice therapy is regarded by the majority of speech pathologists in Israel as a small professional niche.

ISHLA has not yet established clinical practice guidelines for voice evaluation or voice therapy. Therefore clinical practice varies from clinic to clinic. There is a general consensus among most voice therapists in Israel that voice evaluation should be multidimensional and that it should be based on a variety of assessment tools. However, in clinical practice most clinicians rely on a non-standardised perceptual evaluation of voice and vocal behaviour alone. Only a small number of clinicians incorporate acoustic analysis, listeners' rating scales, self-evaluation questionnaires or aerodynamic measurements in their routine assessment protocol. Indeed, the majority of ENT and speech pathology professionals consider perceptual voice evaluation as the gold standard, while all other evaluation options are considered as supplementary, useful only for research but not for clinical purposes.

## Acoustic analysis

Over past years, a number of developments have been observed among the Israeli voice clinicians. For example, some centres have included acoustic analysis of voice as part of the routine evaluation of voice disorders. Computer programs such as Praat© (Boersma & Weenink, 2011) or KayPentax's

Multi-Dimensional Voice Program (MDVP™; Kay-Pentax) have been used in the evaluation and therapeutic processes. Consequently, normative data on the acoustic properties of voice among Hebrew speakers have become available (e.g. Amir et al., 2009), for clinical use.

## Perceptual voice evaluation

Perceptual evaluation of voice quality is considered the gold standard for clinical voice evaluation (e.g. Yu et al., 2002). However, in Israel the use of a non-standardised approach for perceptual voice evaluation and the use of different terminologies present difficulties in communication among the professionals. Clinical bias in voice evaluation also makes it difficult for comparison across centres. With the inherent limitation of non-standardised perceptual voice evaluation in mind, the voice profession has attempted to adopt standardised procedures. The GRBAS scale (Hirano, 1981) has become a popular rating scale in recent years despite criticism about it (e.g. Bhuta et al., 2004). The CAPE-V (Karnell et al., 2007) is another standardised tool used in some Israeli clinics, though it seems that the majority of clinicians who incorporate perceptual rating scales into their clinical routine work prefer using the GRBAS. It should be noted that neither of these two scales has been translated, modified or standardised for the Hebrew population.

## Voice-related quality of life measurement

The patients' self-evaluation of the voice problem has received increasing attention over the past 20 years. Two of these tools that have been standardised in English have been translated and adapted for use in Hebrew. They are the Voice Handicap Index (VHI) and its shortened version, the VHI-10 (Amir et al., 2006a, 2006b). These tools are now used in some clinics as part of the standardised protocol of the preliminary voice evaluation. Another self-evaluation questionnaire, the Voice-Related Quality of Life (V-RQOL; Karnell et al., 2007), has also been translated and adapted for use in Hebrew. However, the Hebrew version of V-RQOL has not been published and therefore is not commonly used in clinical practice.

# Additional Issues Related to Voice Therapy in Israel

## Paediatric voice cases

Voice therapy in Israel is mainly financially covered by the public health system. A maximum of 12 therapy sessions can be given, based on a recommendation made by an ENT physician or a family practitioner. The minimum age for enrolling in voice therapy is not officially defined, and the majority of clinicians in Israel would typically prefer not to enrol children under the age of 7–8 years. Nevertheless, more clinicians now recognise that age is not the only factor that should be considered in accepting patients for voice therapy. Other factors include the child's ability to tolerate a laryngeal examination, awareness of his/her voice problem, motivation, compliance and cooperation, as well as the parents' expectation and compliance.

While voice therapy for adults is mostly performed in clinics, voice therapy for children can be conducted in school or at the child's home, either on an individual basis or in small groups. The duration of the treatment in the public system is similar to that for adults.

## Preventive voice therapy

Preventive voice therapy is another area in which voice clinicians are routinely involved in Israel. Colleges require student teachers to participate in a preventive voice workshop during their studies. It is believed that educating future teachers to take care of their voices in order to prevent the development of voice disorders is more cost-effective than providing them with voice therapy when it is needed. These preventive workshops provide the students with basic knowledge about the vocal mechanism and vocal hygiene education as well as basic breathing and voicing exercises.

Between 1996 and 1999, the Department of Communication Disorders at Tel-Aviv University conducted a community project for the prevention of voice problems among schoolteachers. The 241 teachers who completed the 14-session program and participated in the follow-up session (6 months post-therapy) reported a significant improvement in their voice quality, and a significant *reduction* in vocal complaints. In addition, teachers who only participated in the opening lecture of the project but did not participate in the 14 sessions (N = 58) also reported a reduction in the number of vocal complaints (Muchnik *et al.*, 2001). This project shows the usefulness of preventive voice therapy for future teachers.

# Future Directions

The number of speech pathologists in Israel interested in voice disorders is still small. This number would not be sufficient to generate a critical mass in order to facilitate developments in voice assessment or therapy areas. It therefore seems appropriate for the initial goal to be to find a means to increase clinicians' interest in voice. The second goal is to further develop culturally sensitive diagnostic and treatment tools for the diverse and multilingual population of Israel. This will of course require collaboration among the different medical centres in Israel, and between Israeli clinicians and scientists, as well as the international professional community. Finally, although it seems that most voice clinicians in Israel are up-to-date on the advances in the fields of voice and voice therapy, this is not always reflected in the infrastructure found in the clinical setting. New therapeutic approaches, multidimensional evaluation of voice and other advances in the field should be incorporated into clinical settings and practice, and should not just be restricted to the research field. This goal could probably be achieved through collaboration between the Israeli academia and ISHLA. Such collaboration could be in the form of joint research and developing advanced studies for clinicians who are interested in advancing their theoretical knowledge and clinical skills in the field of voice science and disorders.

## References

Amir, O. (2011) Voice therapy for children and adolescents. Paper presented at the World Voice Day Symposium, 8 April, Tel-Hashomer, Israel.

Amir, O., Ashkenazi, O., Leibovitzh, T., Michael, O., Tavor, Y. and Wolf, M. (2006a) Applying the Voice Handicap Index (VHI) to dysphonic and nondysphonic Hebrew speakers. *Journal of Voice* 20, 318–324.

Amir, O., Tavor, Y., Leibovitzh, T., Ashkenazi, O., Michael, O., Primov-Fever, A., *et al.* (2006b) Evaluating the validity of the Voice Handicap Index-10 (VHI-10) among Hebrew speakers. *Otolaryngology – Head and Neck Surgery* 135 (4), 603–607.

Amir, O., Wolf, M. and Amir, N. (2009) A clinical comparison between two acoustic analysis softwares: MDVP and Praat. *Biomedical Signal Processing and Control* 4, 202–205.

Bhuta, T., Patrick, L. and Garnett, J.D. (2004) Perceptual evaluation of voice quality and its correlation with acoustic measurements. *Journal of Voice* 18, 299–304.

Boersma, P. and Weenink, D. (2011) Praat: doing phonetics by computer (Version 5.2.19) [computer program], accessed 16 March 2011. http://www.praat.org/

Hirano, M. (1981) Psycho-acoustic evaluation of voice: GRBAS scale for evaluating the hoarse voice. In M. Hirano (ed.) *Clinical Examination of Voice* (pp. 81–84). Vienna: Springer.

Karnell, M.P., Melton, S.D., Childes, J.M., Coleman, T.C., Dailey, S.A. and Hoffman, H.T. (2007) Reliability of clinician-based (GRBAS and CAPE-V) and patient-based (V-RQOL and IPVI) documentation of voice disorders. *Journal of Voice* 21, 576–590.

Laguaite, J.K. (1972) Adult voice screening. *Journal of Speech and Hearing Disorders* 37, 147–151.

Morley, D.E. (1952) A ten-year survey of speech disorders among university students. *Journal of Speech and Hearing Disorders* 17, 25–31.

Muchnik, C., Hertzberg, O., Mekai, E., Shabtai, E., Yedwab, D., Ezrati, R., *et al.* (2001) A community project for prevention of voice disorders among school teachers: 1996–1999. *Seeing the Voices – Cathedra for Professional Publications in the Field of Hearing Impairments* 1, 66–72 [in Hebrew].

Yu, P., Revis J., Wuyts, F.L., Zanaret, M. and Giovanni, A. (2002) Correlation of instrumental voice evaluation with perceptual voice analysis using a modified visual analog scale. *Folia Phoniatrica et Logopedica* 54, 271–281.

# 7 Contemporary Phonosurgery in Japan

## Koichi Tsunoda

### History of Phonosurgery in Japan

Based on the results of a PubMed search, the word 'phonosurgery' was first published in a Spanish article in 1971 (Von Leden, 1971), and subsequently Isshiki used it in the first report in English in 1980 (Isshiki, 1980). Many Japanese laryngologists have contributed a great deal to the conducted research on laryngeal anatomy, physiology and pathology and have attempted to utilize the results to develop original phonosurgical procedures.

Saito (1966) developed and established the basis of the current phonomicrosurgery known as laryngomicrosurgery in the 1960s. His report was first published in Japanese (Saito, 1966). Laryngomicrosurgery became widespread in Japan and now refers to any type of phonosurgery for the removal of vocal fold polyps, nodules, Rainke's edema, cysts and benign or malignant lesions, and for vocal fold augmentation for glottal incompetence.

Another important development was laryngeal framework surgery, which was developed by Isshiki and colleagues (1974, 1978) in an effort to resolve other laryngeal problems that could not be treated successfully with laryngomicrosurgery. In particular, the thyroplasty type-1 and arytenoid rotation techniques were evolved for the treatment of glottal incompetence (Isshiki et al., 1974). These framework and medialization techniques were subsequently adopted worldwide and referred to as the 'Isshiki procedures'. Tokashiki et al. (2005) developed an additional natural approach for medialization using the lateral cricoarytenoid (LCA) muscle.

Japanese phonosurgeons continue to devise novel approaches for the treatment of difficult vocal problems, modified previously established surgical techniques to make them less invasive and succeeded in developing appropriate solutions for some problematic conditions. One of those solutions was fiber optic laryngeal surgery under local anesthesia. In 1965, the Research Institute of Logopedics and Phoniatrics was established within the Faculty of Medicine of the University of Tokyo, where Sawashima and

Hirose (1968) developed and established the flexible laryngeal fiberscope for laryngeal examination. In the early 1990s, for example, Hesaka and colleagues first performed intracordal atelocollagen injection to treat glottal incompetence caused by unilateral laryngeal paralysis under local anesthesia using a flexible fiberscope and a stroboscope with a video monitoring system (Hesaka *et al.*, 1994). Omori and colleagues (2000) introduced flexible videoendoscope-assisted laryngeal surgery through the nasal cavity with office-based equipment. In this technique, the patient remains seated while the nose, pharynx and larynx are topically anesthetized in an outpatient surgical procedure (Omori *et al.*, 2000).

Since only a small forceps tip can pass through a fiberscope channel, a limited range of forceps was originally available for use in fiberscope procedures. In phonosurgery, in cases where it is not possible to use a rigid laryngoscope, a flexible fiberscope with laryngeal-mask ventilation may be used (Kikkawa *et al.*, 2004). As a solution to those problems, a detachable forceps was developed for flexible fiber optic surgery (Tsunoda *et al.*, 2002a).

Although the original Japanese laryngomicrosurgery, framework surgical techniques and advances in fiber optic surgery contributed to resolving many issues in phonosurgery, other problems remain. Two such problems are pathological sulcus vocalis resulting from scar formation and spasmodic dysphonia. This chapter reviews the current challenges and describes less invasive, safe, effective techniques used in Japan to treat difficult cases.

## Traditional treatment for glottal incompetence

Many methods have been reported for the treatment of glottal incompetence. Behavioral voice therapies for glottal incompetence were generally attempted before surgical intervention (Tsunoda *et al.*, 2003; Yamaguchi *et al.*, 1993). Previously, the aim of surgical treatment reported by most researchers was to produce adequate glottal closure during phonation. Surgical methods to improve glottal closure have used vocal fold augmentation techniques (injections) or laryngeal framework surgery.

### Vocal fold augmentation techniques (injections)

Arnold's procedure for vocal fold augmentation became the global standard (Arnold, 1962). Rubin (1965) introduced silicone as a new material for vocal fold injection, and silicone has been used widely in Japan since that report. Fukuda and colleagues (1970) introduced this technique for vocal rehabilitation in Japan. They compared solid and liquid types of silicone implants in their experimental research and identified the characteristic differences between the two types of silicones clinically. Liquid implants are ultimately absorbed and therefore useful for temporary vocal improvement in patients in whom the prognosis for vocal paralysis is not known. On the other hand, solid implants are not absorbed and therefore are effective in the long term when spontaneous vocal fold recovery can be ruled out (Tsuzuki *et al.*, 1991).

Bovine collagen injections have also been widely used as an alternative to alloplastic materials (Ford & Bless, 1986; Ford *et al.*, 1992). However, because bioimplants such as bovine collagen are foreign substances, an alternative is the transplantation of autologous tissue into the vocal fold. Around 1990, autologous lipoinjection (Mikaelian *et al.*, 1991) and autologous fat (Brandenburg *et al.*, 1992) injection began to be performed in cases of glottal incompetence. Around the same time, bovine spongiform encephalopathy (BSE) became an issue of great concern worldwide (Aldhous, 1990; Lancet, 1988, 1990). In light of the medicosocial concerns about BSE, it became clear that autologous materials were preferable to other options for injection into the vocal folds. Concerns about the possibility of allergic responses have also limited the clinical use of bovine collagen, and therefore autologous fat (Brandenburg *et al.*, 1992; Mikaelian *et al.*, 1991), collagen (Ford *et al.*, 1995) and fascia (Rihkanen, 1998) injections were introduced. In cases where fat injection is indicated, Tamura and colleagues (2008) reported the use of autologous buccal instead of abdominal fat injection with successful results (Tamura *et al.*, 2010).

It now appears clear that, in vocal fold augmentation to treat glottal incompetence, autologous materials are preferable to alloplastic or (heterologous) bioimplant materials for injection into the vocal folds. In addition to being safer, they are less likely to be rejected and are more likely to remain stable for longer periods.

### Laryngeal framework surgery

Isshiki and co-workers developed the basic technique of medialization thyroplasty as a type of framework surgery at the beginning of the 1970s (Isshiki *et al.*, 1974). To correct glottal incompetence caused by unilateral vocal fold paralysis, the Isshiki type-I technique or the alternative arytenoid-adduction procedure (Isshiki *et al.*, 1978) has been widely adopted worldwide.

## Problems in the traditional treatment of sulcus vocalis

In the past, injections of bovine collagen in both vocal folds were administered to achieve satisfactory glottal closure and to prevent breathy phonation in cases of sulcus vocalis. After surgery, the glottal chink disappeared and the maximum phonation time (MPT) increased. However, this improvement often lasted for only a few months. Because this technique uses synthetic material or foreign tissue and because the beneficial effects are not sustained for a sufficiently long period, we thought it was necessary to develop a new type of surgery.

Based on clinical observations, Tsunoda and colleagues (1997a, 1997b) hypothesized that, even if surgery affected both Reinke's space and the superficial layer of the lamina propria, the epithelium and lamina propria might be renewed after 6 months to 1 year. Taking into account the emerging research into stem cell transplantation (Tsubota, 1997), it seemed likely that stem cells would contribute to those improvements. Stem cells or stem cell-like functional cells might be able to proliferate within this area.

## Earlier attempts for the treatment of sulcus vocalis

Our hypothesis on the development of new tissue led us to attempt a previously untried surgical approach for the treatment of sulcus vocalis. First, we made a lateral incision in the surface of the vocal fold epithelium to separate the sulcus from the vocal fold ligament. Then we dissected the surface from the body to a depth of 3 mm below the sulcus. Finally, we injected bovine collagen into the body of the vocal fold. The results of our new separation and injection procedure were not satisfactory. However, they were indeed similar to the results of previous collagen injections.

An idea for a suitable injection material arose from our experience with otological surgery. Specifically, the temporal fascia had been used successfully by otologists in performing tympanoplasty. This fascia, which forms a covering layer over the temporalis muscle, is composed of the appropriate type of tissue for the repair of vocal fold pathology and might include healthy cells that could undergo proliferation. Furthermore, the transplantation of the fascia does not involve synthetic materials or foreign tissues. We therefore assumed that it would carry a low risk of infection and be immunologically safe. Finally, we had developed a completely different approach to the treatment of pathological sulcus vocalis, which not only achieves the vocal fold augmentation but also improves vocalization. This new procedure is known as autologous transplantation of the fascia into the vocal fold (ATFV; Figure 7.1) (Tsunoda & Niimi, 2000; Tsunoda et al., 1999, 2001, 2005a).

Since 1997 we have performed the ATFV procedure to treat patients with sulcus vocalis. The long-term results of our new surgical approach and the role of this type of transplantation are summarized and discussed below (Tsunoda et al., 2001, 2005a).

(1) Six months after ATFV, the MPT gradually increased and stroboscopy showed consistently improved glottal closure. Six months to 1 year after transplantation, further improvement was noted.

(2) One year after surgery, stroboscopy showed excellent glottal closure, including satisfactory mucosal waves during phonation. Hyperadduction of the ventricular folds also disappeared in all our patients.

(3) Three years after surgery, improvement of the MPT, presence of mucosal waves and normal adduction of the ventricular folds remained at excellent levels.

(4) We have not seen any critical complications after performing ATFV (after adjustments to resolve short-term complications). Because the transplantation is autologous, complications associated with immunological reactions do not occur.

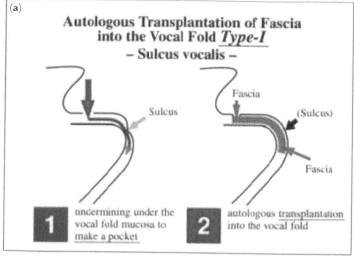

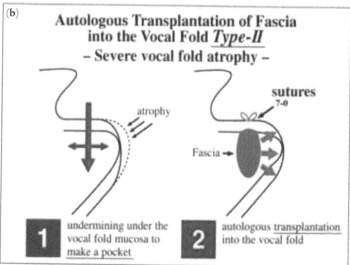

**Figure 7.1** (a–d) Surgical approaches in phonosurgery

(5)   ATFV can induce the production and proliferation of the extracellular matrix and thus may be one of the most logical therapeutic procedures for correcting sulcus vocalis or scarred vocal folds.

Although ATFV was confirmed to be effective in treating pathological sulcus vocalis, the disadvantage is that 6–12 months are required to resolve vocal problems completely because it is a type of regenerative surgery. To improve vocal function immediately after surgery, Nishiyama et al. (2002)

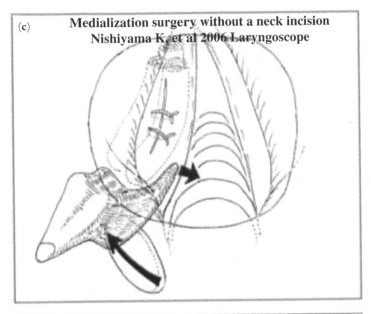

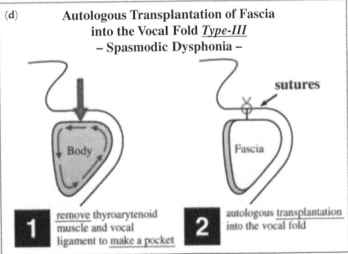

**Figure 7.1** *Continued*

modified the ATFV procedure by employing rolled-up fascia with a much greater volume transplanted and achieved successful results even for unilateral vocal fold paralysis. In addition, Kishimoto's group used a collagen sponge impregnated with growth factor to improve the regeneration of scarred vocal folds including pathological sulcus (Kishimoto *et al.*, 2009).

It is likely that ATFV will continue to play a role in gene therapy and tissue engineering development in the future. Furthermore, ATFV has provided a platform for the establishment of advanced new phonosurgical techniques (autologous transplantation, separation of the epithelium, suturing of the epithelium) known collectively as phonoultramicrosurgery (Fujii & Tsunoda, 2008).

## Combination and modification of Isshiki's procedure for vocal fold paralysis

Generally, Isshiki's medialization technique is performed in cases of glottal incompetence caused by unilateral vocal fold paralysis. A main advantage of this technique is that it is possible to adjust the vertical level of both vocal processes. However, if the glottal incompetence is caused by paralysis, vocal fold atrophy will remain even after successful surgery. There are reports on how to improve voice quality and atrophy in the literature. In particular, unilateral laryngeal nerve paralysis occurs in some patients with thyroid carcinoma. Ansa hypoglossi-recurrent laryngeal nerve anastomosis was a traditional technique for the prevention of vocal fold atrophy after unilateral vocal fold paralysis (Crumley & Izdebski, 1986). To restore the tonus of the immobile vocal fold, Tucker described nerve-muscle pedicle (NMP) flap implantation onto the thyroarytenoid (TA) muscle through the window in the thyroid ala (May & Beery, 1986; Tucker, 1976). NMP implantations were performed onto the TA muscle (Tucker, 1976) or LCA muscle (May & Beery, 1986) in such cases.

Yumoto's group performed studies in animals (Miyamaru et al., 2009) and experimented clinically with reinnervation of the vocal folds. Finally, they developed an arytenoid adduction surgical technique combined with NMP flap implantation with successful results (Yumoto et al., 2010). Their technique can be summarized as follows: The omohyoid muscle is transected, and the ansa cervicalis (AC) nerve is followed until it enters the sternohyoid (SH) muscle. Electrical stimulation is applied to confirm the presence of nerve fibers innervating the SH muscle. A relatively thick AC branch to the SH muscle is harvested together with a 3 × 3-mm section of muscle at the point of nerve entrance to the muscle to form an NMP flap.

Arytenoid adduction is performed following the usual approach, with 3-0 nylon sutures securing the muscular process. A window is drilled in the thyroid ala, the perichondrium is excised with electrocautery and the TA muscle is carefully exposed as widely as possible to secure contact of the NMP flap with the TA muscle. Then the nylon sutures holding the muscular process in place are introduced on the anterior surface of the thyroid ala medially from the inferior tubercle, with one end passing through the lower edge of the window and the other end through the cricothyroid membrane. Then the muscle section of the NMP flap is positioned in the window to form as wide a contact as possible with the TA muscle and secured to the surrounding tissues using 8-0 nylon sutures. Finally, the window is covered with the outer perichondrium. Yumoto's new technique can be modified not only to treat glottal incompetence and adjust the vertical level of both vocal folds, but also to improve the tonus of paralyzed vocal folds.

# A less invasive approach to treating vocal fold lesions

In the past two decades, many forms of surgery have been modified to less invasive procedures under general anesthesia. Phonosurgery has also been converted from requiring a skin incision in the neck to techniques without a skin incision. In cases of unilateral vocal fold paralysis resulting from thorax, cardiac, pulmonary or thyroid surgery, some patients refused further skin incisions in the neck which would result in visible scarring, even when reassured that arytenoid rotation or thyroplasty could improve the vocal fold paralysis. As a result, the injection of collagen or autologous fat was performed in these patients using laryngomicrosurgery. Although such injections are less invasive, the results are not as satisfactory as those of medialization surgeries. However, patients still preferred to have their hoarseness treated without surgery under general anesthesia. Clinic-based injections using laryngeal fiber optic phonosurgical techniques (Hesaka et al., 1994; Omori et al., 2000) were therefore advantageous for such patients as well as for outpatient treatment of nodules and polyps.

## Modified medialization surgery without neck incision

Injection laryngoplasty is another procedure for treating unilateral vocal fold paralysis. Sato and colleagues performed lipoinjections in three patients with the endolaryngeal microsurgical technique under general anesthesia (Sato et al., 2004). The locations of fat injections were the vocal fold, ventricular fold, aryepiglottic fold of the larynx and medial wall of the pyriform sinus of the hypopharynx. Lipoinjection into the vocal fold, ventricular fold and aryepiglottic fold strengthen laryngeal closure. Lipoinjection into the TA muscle lateral to the oblong fovea of the arytenoid cartilage enables arytenoid cartilage rotation and consequently strengthens laryngeal closure. Sato et al. (2004) concluded that modified injection laryngoplasty (laryngohypopharyngoplasty) is one surgical option for preventing aspiration after vocal fold paralysis.

ATFV is also effective in treating cases of unilateral vocal fold paralysis, using type-2 autologous transplantation for minimal glottal chinks. However, the results of ATFV are not satisfactory in patients with severe glottal chinks. It was therefore necessary to combine ATFV type-2 (to resolve the atrophy) and arytenoid rotation (for abduction of the vocal process) to resolve severe glottal chinks. When we were attempting to develop this combined surgical technique, we treated an interesting case of pseudo-vocal-cord paralysis in a patient who had swallowed a fish bone (Tsunoda *et al.*, 2002). The fish bone had become wedged between the arytenoid cartilage and thyroid cartilage, causing unilateral vocal process rotation around the physiologically median position as a result of constriction of the LCA muscle. The bone was removed by laryngomicrosurgery without complications. Based on their experience in treating that patient and after careful review of the anatomy and physiology of the case, Nishiyama *et al.* (2005) reported successful results using an ATFV technique for medialization surgery without a neck incision. The long-term results were also satisfactory (Nishiyama *et al.*, 2006). Ikeda and co-workers (2006) considered calcium phosphate cement (CPC) for laryngeal injection and found that the focal foreign body reaction to injected CPC was almost the same as that to autologous fat. Shiotani *et al.* (2009) have recently performed successful medialization surgery with CPC injection. Even in patients with a large posterior glottal gap, CPC can be injected into the lateral side of the ipsilateral vocal process to adduct the arytenoid cartilage (Shiotani *et al.*, 2009). These new types of medialization surgery were performed using the laryngomicrosurgery technique under general anesthesia without a neck incision.

## A solution for abduction-type spasmodic dysphonia

Currently, one of the difficult problems facing laryngeal surgeons is the treatment of adduction-type spasmodic dysphonia (AdSD). Dedo (1976) performed recurrent laryngeal-nerve resection. However, his long-term results showed that approximately 80% of nerve-section patients considered their voices to be too weak for adequate communication in noisy environments at the fourth postoperative year. Hoarseness occurred because of the resulting unilateral recurrent laryngeal-nerve paralysis, and significant persistent breathiness occurred in 10–15% of patients (Dedo & Izdebski, 1983). To prevent breathy hoarseness, Iwamura *et al.* (1979) performed selective resection of a branch of the recurrent laryngeal nerve (i.e. the branch to the TA muscle) to treat spasmodic dysphonia.

Botulinum toxin (Botox) injection (Miller *et al.*, 1987) has also been performed in Japan by Kobayashi and his associates since the early 1990s (Kobayashi *et al.*, 1993). In general, patients with AdSD experience stress (physiological and psychological) when scheduled to receive botulinum toxin injections four times per year. They demanded a more effective procedure with more consistent, longer lasting results and also expressed concern about being injected with a 'toxin'. Isshiki developed four laryngeal framework surgical techniques (thyroplasty types 1–4; Isshiki *et al.*, 1974); one technique (type 3, the anterior-posterior shortening of the thyroid ala to relax vocal fold tension) was found to be effective in treating AdSD (Isshiki, 1989).

The disadvantages of previous surgical techniques to treat AdSD can be summarized as follows: (1) after nerve resection or myectomy, hoarseness occurred because of permanent unilateral recurrent laryngeal-nerve paralysis and/or vocal fold atrophy; (2) framework surgery is highly invasive and requires a surgical incision on the anterior surface of the patient's neck; (3) the beneficial effects of botulinum toxin injection last for only a few months and therefore patients must receive an injection every 3 months.

Ono et al. (1998) reported a new type of surgery to treat spasmodic dys-phonia, where part of the vocalis muscle is removed and the defective section is replaced with fibrinogen glue (Tisseel®). This procedure is effective in resolving spastic voice (Ono et al., 1998), but it can also result in glottal incompetence. Breathy hoarseness gradually resolves within 6 months after the surgery. Based on the biophysical mora method, improved vocalization was noted in all seven patients evaluated (Nakamura et al., 2008).

Isshiki's type-3 thyroplasty procedure is theoretically an effective way to decrease the hypertensive adduction of the vocal folds. However, it is very invasive in comparison with botulinum toxin injection. Based on previous experience, botulinum toxin injections are effective even when administered only unilaterally. Therefore we replaced the body of the unilateral vocal fold using the ATFV type-2 approach to treat AdSD (Tsunoda & Niimi, 2000). First, the vocalis muscle, TA muscle and vocal ligament are removed. Finally, the vocal fold body is replaced with an autologous fascia temporalis-like type-2 ATFV transplantation (Tsunoda et al., 2005b).

Isshiki and colleagues reported using a midline type-2 thyroplasty (lat-eralization) procedure for AdSD (Isshiki & Sanuki, 2010; Isshiki et al., 2004), using a titanium bridge in place of a silicone shim. Successful long-term results were also reported (Sanuki & Isshiki, 2007). This new Isshiki proce-dure, which requires a neck incision, may be the most effective phonosurgi-cal approach to date. Isshiki and colleagues continuously analyzed their surgical outcomes objectively and then developed solutions for any short-comings in the technique used. The use of a titanium bridge in place of a silicone shim was found to be essential in the midline type-2 thyroplasty for AdSD (Isshiki & Sanuki, 2010; Sanuki & Isshiki, 2009). Although it is necessary to consider the indications carefully and surgeons must be skilled, this new Isshiki type-2 procedure using the titanium bridge may be the most effective phonosurgical approach for the treatment of AdSD involving a neck incision.

## Tissue engineering and future therapy

The ultimate objective of phonosurgery is to improve the voice to the degree desired by patients. Based on the successful results of experimental animal studies, Omori and colleagues (2005) demonstrated regeneration of the tracheal tissue using an in situ tissue engineering technique for airway reconstruction in the first human example of the repair of the trachea in thyroid cancer. A Marlex mesh tube covered by a collagen sponge was used as a tissue scaffold. Good epithelialization has been observed on the tracheal luminal surface without any complications during a 2-year follow-up. Although long-term follow-up is necessary, regenerative therapy of the tracheal tissue appears feasible for airway reconstruction (Omori et al., 2005). After further animal studies, Omori's group established the clinical application of in situ tissue engineering using a scaffolding technique for airway defects (Omori et al., 2008). They have refined the tissue scaffold made from a Marlex mesh tube covered by a collagen sponge, and in situ tissue engineering with a scaffold implant was employed to repair the larynx and trachea in three patients with thyroid cancer. The trachea and cricoid cartilage with tumor invasion were resected, and the scaffold was implanted into the tissue. Postoperative endoscopy during follow-up periods of 8–34 months showed well-epithelialized airway lumens without obstruction (Omori et al., 2008).

Hirano and colleagues (2008) first reported the therapeutic potential of basic fibroblast growth factor (bFGF) for tissue regeneration of the aged vocal fold in a 63-year-old man. Atrophy of the vocal fold improved 1 week after bFGF injection, and the glottal gap disappeared. Aerodynamic and acoustic parameters also showed marked improvement. These effects were maintained for up to 3 months. The results are encouraging, suggesting that the therapeutic effects of bFGF could be applied to treat atrophied vocal folds in humans (Hirano et al., 2008). Those new developments were established based on traditional animal studies, as reported in a previous chapter.

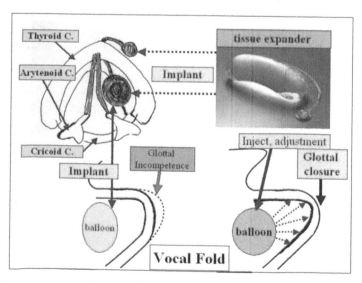

**Figure 7.2** Proposed artificial vocal fold construction

Tissue engineering with autologous cells or tissues appears to be the most appropriate method for the repair of pathological conditions. Another pre-developmental surgical technique is artificial laryngeal structures. A new concept for an artificial vocal fold structure is introduced here for the consideration of phonosurgeons (Tsunoda, 2009). Anti-aging devices and procedures to improve hearing (e.g. hearing aids, cochlear implants) and vision (e.g. eyeglasses, intraocular lenses) are well established as communication support tools in the 'speech chain'. They can be fitted to individual needs and adjusted as those needs change. However, tools to improve vocal problems associated with physiological aging are not as well established. Considering previous phonosurgical techniques against the background of my experience, I would like to propose a completely different approach to the treatment of glottal incompetence. I suggest a new adjustable surgical technique to replace injection therapies. The proposed solution is implanting an inflatable bag or balloon on the lateral side of the vocal fold (Figure 7.2). Unlike ATFV procedures, where the implanted material appears to become vocal fold tissue, the new implant would function as an artificial vocal fold. In the future, using this proposed technique, the degree of augmentation can be adjusted to meet changing physical conditions.

## References

Aldhous, P. (1990) BSE. No madness in UK policy. *Nature* 346 (6281), 211.

Arnold, G. (1962) Vocal rehabilitation of paralytic dysphonia: VIII. Phoniatric methods of vocal compensation. *Archives of Otolaryngology – Head and Neck Surgery* 76, 76–83.

Brandenburg, J., Kirkham, W. and Koschkee, D. (1992) Vocal cord augmentation with autogenous fat. *Laryngoscope* 102 (5), 495–500.

Crumley, R. and Izdebski, K. (1986) Voice quality following laryngeal reinnervation by ansa hypoglossi transfer. *Laryngoscope* 96 (6), 611–616.

Dedo, H. (1976) Recurrent laryngeal nerve section for spastic dysphonia. *Annals of Otology, Rhinology, and Laryngology* 85 (4:1), 451–459.

Dedo, H. and Izdebski, K. (1983) Intermediate results of 306 recurrent laryngeal nerve sections for spastic dysphonia. *Laryngoscope* 93 (1), 9–16.

Ford, C. and Bless, D. (1986) A preliminary study of injectable collagen in human vocal fold augmentation. *Otolaryngology – Head and Neck Surgery* 94 (1), 104–122.

Ford, C., Bless, D. and Loftus, J. (1992) Role of injectable collagen in the treatment of glottic insufficiency: A study of 119 patients. *Annals of Otology, Rhinology, and Laryngology* 101 (3), 237–247.

Ford, C., Staskowski, P. and Bless, D. (1995) Autologous collagen vocal fold injection: A preliminary clinical study. *Laryngoscope* 105 (9), 944–948.

Fujii, R. and Tsunoda, K. (2008) Safe, complete resection of epiglottic cysts with phono-ultra-microsurgical technique. *Journal of Laryngology and Otology* 122 (2), 201–203.

Fukuda, H. (1970) Vocal rehabilitation using injectable silicone. *Nippon Jibiinkoka Gakkai Kaiho* 73 (9), 1506–1526.

Hesaka, H., Miyano, R., Matsui, M., Kamide, Y. and Moriyama, H. (1994) Intracordal injection therapy using atelocollagen for unilateral laryngeal paralysis under local anesthesia. *Nippon Jibiinkoka Gakkai Kaiho* 97 (5), 847–854.

Hirano, S., Kishimoto, Y., Suehiro, A., Kanemaru, S. and Ito, J. (2008) Regeneration of aged vocal fold: First human case treated with fibroblast growth factor. *Laryngoscope* 118 (12), 2254–2259.

Ikeda, A., Shiotani, A., Mori, Y., Fujimine, T., Tomifuji, M., Takaoka, T., *et al.* (2006) Suitability of calcium phosphate cement for injection laryngoplasty in rabbits. *Journal for Oto-Rhino-Laryngology and its Related Specialties* 68 (2), 103–109.

Isshiki, N. (1980) Recent advances in phonosurgery. *Folia Phoniatrica et Logopaedica* 32 (2), 119–154.

Isshiki, N. (1989) *Phonosurgery: Theory and Practice* (pp. 1–233). Tokyo: Springer-Verlag.

Isshiki, N. and Sanuki, T. (2010) Surgical tips for type II thyroplasty for adductor spasmodic dysphonia: Modified technique after reviewing unsatisfactory cases. *Acta Oto-laryngologica* 130 (2), 275–280.

Isshiki, N., Morita, H., Okamura, H. and Hiramoto, M. (1974) Thyroplasty as a new phonosurgical technique. *Acta Oto-laryngologica* 78 (1–6), 451–457.

Isshiki, N., Tanabe, M. and Sawada, M. (1978) Arytenoid adduction for unilateral vocal cord paralysis. *Archives of Otolaryngology – Head and Neck Surgery* 104 (10), 555–558.

Isshiki, N., Yamamoto, I. and Fukagai, S. (2004) Type 2 thyroplasty for spasmodic dysphonia: Fixation using a titanium bridge. *Acta Oto-laryngologica* 124 (3), 309–312.

Iwamura, S., Yajima, K. and Hirose, H. (1979) Selective section of thyroarytenoid branch of recurrent laryngeal nerve. *Nippon Jibiinkoka Gakkai Kaiho* 82, 1046–1047.

Kikkawa, Y., Tsunoda, K. and Niimi, S. (2004) Prediction and surgical management of difficult laryngoscopy. *Laryngoscope* 114 (4), 776–778.

Kishimoto, Y., Hirano, S., Kojima, T., Kanemaru, S. and Ito, J. (2009) Implantation of an atelocollagen sheet for the treatment of vocal fold scarring and sulcus vocalis. *Annals of Otology, Rhinology & Laryngology* 118 (9), 613–620.

Kobayashi, T., Niimi, S., Kumada, M., Kosaki, H. and Hirose, H. (1993) Botulinum toxin treatment for spasmodic dysphonia. *Acta Oto-laryngologica* 113 (S504), 155–157.

Lancet (1988) BSE and scrapie: agent for change. *Lancet* 2, 607–608.

Lancet (1990) BSE in perspective. *Lancet* 335, 1252–1253.

May, M. and Beery, Q. (1986) Muscle-nerve pedicle laryngeal reinnervation. *Laryngoscope* 96 (11), 1196–1200.

Mikaelian, D., Lowry, L. and Sataloff, R. (1991) Lipoinjection for unilateral vocal cord paralysis. *Laryngoscope* 101 (5), 465–468.

Miller, R., Woodson, G. and Jankovic, J. (1987) Botulinum toxin injection of the vocal fold for spasmodic dysphonia: A preliminary report. *Archives of Otolaryngology – Head and Neck Surgery* 113 (6), 603–605.

Miyamaru, S., Kumai, Y., Ito, T., Sanuki, T. and Yumoto, E. (2009) Nerve-muscle pedicle implantation facilitates re-innervation of long-term denervated thyroarytenoid muscle in rats. *Acta Oto-laryngologica* 129 (12), 1486–1492.

Nakamura, K., Muta, H., Watanabe, Y., Mochizuki, R., Yoshida, T. and Suzuki, M. (2008) Surgical treatment for adductor spasmodic dysphonia – efficacy of bilateral thyroarytenoid myectomy under microlaryngoscopy. *Acta Oto-laryngologica* 128 (12), 1348–1353.

Nishiyama, K., Hirose, H., Iguchi, Y., Nagai, H., Yamanaka, J. and Okamoto, M. (2002) Autologous transplantation of fascia into the vocal fold as a treatment for recurrent nerve paralysis. *Laryngoscope* 112 (8), 1420–1425.

Nishiyama, K., Hirose, H., Horiguchi, S. and Tsunoda, K. (2005) Endoscopic vocal cord medialization. *Acta Oto-Laryngolica* 125, 1134–1136.

Nishiyama, K., Hirose, H., Masaki, T., Nagai, H., Hashimoto, D., Usui, D., *et al.* (2006) Long term result of the new endoscopic vocal fold medialization surgical technique for laryngeal palsy. *Laryngoscope* 116 (2), 231–234.

Omori, K., Shinohara, K., Tsuji, T. and Kojima, H. (2000) Videoendoscopic laryngeal surgery. *Annals of Otology, Rhinology, and Laryngology* 109 (2), 149–155.

Omori, K., Nakamura, T., Kanemaru, S., Asato, R., Yamashita, M., Tanaka, S., *et al.* (2005) Regenerative medicine of the trachea: The first human case. *Annals of Otology, Rhinology & Laryngology* 114 (6), 429–433.

Omori, K., Tada, Y., Suzuki, T., Nomoto, Y., Matsuzuka, T., Kobayashi, K., *et al.* (2008) Clinical application of in situ tissue engineering using a scaffolding technique for reconstruction of the larynx and trachea. *Annals of Otology, Rhinology & Laryngology* 117 (9), 673–678.

Ono, J., Muta, H., Mochizuki, R., Tanaka, N., Watanabe, Y. and Kudo, T. (1998) A new surgical treatment for spasmodic dysphonia. *Larynx* 10, 17–21.

Rihkanen, H. (1998) Vocal fold augmentation by injection of autologous fascia. *Laryngoscope* 108 (1), 51–54.

Rubin, H. (1965) Intracordal injection of silicone in selected dysphonias. *Archives of Otolaryngology – Head and Neck Surgery* 81 (6), 604–607.

Saito, S. (1966) Endoscopic microsurgery of the larynx. *Journal of the Japan Broncho-Esophagological Society* 17, 253–266.

Sanuki, T. and Isshiki, N. (2007) Overall evaluation of effectiveness of type II thyroplasty for adductor spasmodic dysphonia. *Laryngoscope* 117 (12), 2255–2259.

Sanuki, T. and Isshiki, N. (2009) Outcomes of type II thyroplasty for adductor spasmodic dysphonia: Analysis of revision and unsatisfactory cases. *Acta Oto-laryngologica* 129 (11), 1287–1293.

Sato, K., Umeno, H. and Nakashima, T. (2004) Autologous fat injection laryngohypopha-ryngoplasty for aspiration after vocal fold paralysis. *Annals of Otology, Rhinology, and Laryngology* 113 (2), 87–92.

Sawashima, M. and Hirose, H. (1968) New laryngoscopic technique by use of fiber optics. *Journal of the Acoustical Society of America* 43, 168–169.

Shiotani, A., Okubo, K., Saito, K., Fujimine, T., Tomifuji, M., Ikeda, A., *et al.* (2009) Injection laryngoplasty with calcium phosphate cement. *Otolaryngology – Head and Neck Surgery* 140, 816–821.

Tamura, E., Fukuda, H., Tabata, Y. and Nishimura, M. (2008) Use of the buccal fad pad for vocal cord augmentation. *Acta Oto-laryngologica* 128 (2), 219–224.

Tamura, E., Okada, S., Shibuya, M. and Iida, M. (2010) Comparison of fat tissues used in intracordal autologous fat injection. *Acta Oto-laryngologica* 130 (3), 405–409.

Tokashiki, R., Hiramatsu, H., Tsukahara, K., Yamaguchi, H., Motohashi, R. and Suzuki, M. (2005) Direct pull of lateral cricoarytenoid muscle for unilateral vocal cord paraly-sis. *Acta Oto-laryngologica* 125 (7), 753–758.

Tsubota, K. (1997) Corneal epithelial stem-cell transplantation. *Lancet* 349 (9064), 1556.

Tsunoda, K. (2009) Artificial vocal folds adjustments to a patient's voice as easily as changing hearing aids or eyeglasses. *Medical Hypotheses* 72 (3), 258–260.

Tsunoda, K. and Niimi, S. (2000) Autologous transplantation of fascia into the vocal fold. *Laryngoscope* 110 (4), 680–682.

Tsunoda, K., Nosaka, K., Housui, M., Murano, E., Ishikawa, M. and Imamura, Y. (1997a) A rare case of laryngeal myxoma. *Journal of Laryngology and Otology* 111 (3), 271–273.

Tsunoda, K., Soda, Y., Tojima, H., Shinogami, M., Ohta, Y., Nibu, K., *et al.* (1997b) Stroboscopic observation of the larynx after radiation in patients with T1 glottic carcinoma. *Acta Oto-laryngologica* 117 (S527), 165–166.

Tsunoda, K., Takanosawa, M. and Niimi, S. (1999) Autologous transplantation of fascia into the vocal fold: A new phonosurgical technique for glottal incompetence. *Laryngoscope* 109 (3), 504–508.

Tsunoda, K., Baer, T. and Niimi, S. (2001) Autologous transplantation of fascia into the vocal fold: Long-term results of a new phonosurgical technique for glottal incompe-tence. *Laryngoscope* 111 (3), 453–457.

Tsunoda, K., Kikkawa, Y., Yoshihashi, R. and Sakai, Y. (2002a) Detachable forceps for flexible fibre-optic surgery: A new technique for phonosurgery in cases where rigid laryngoscopy is contraindicated. *Journal of Laryngology and Otology* 116 (07), 559–561.

Tsunoda, K., Sakai, Y., Watanabe, T. and Kikkawa, Y. (2002b) Pseudo vocal cord paralysis caused by a fish bone. *Lancet* 360 (9337), 907.

Tsunoda, K., Kikkawa, Y., Kumada, M., Higo, R. and Tayama, N. (2003) Hoarseness caused by unilateral vocal fold paralysis: How long should one delay phonosurgery? *Acta Oto-laryngologica* 123 (4), 555–556.

Tsunoda, K., Kondou, K., Kaga, K., Niimi, S., Baer, T., Nishiyama, K., *et al.* (2005a) Autologous transplantation of fascia into the vocal fold: Long term result of type 1 transplantation and the future. *Laryngoscope* 115 (S108), 1–10.

Tsunoda, K., Amagai, N., Kondou, K., Baer, T., Kaga, K. and Niimi, S. (2005b) Autologous replacement of the vocal fold: A new surgical approach for adduction-type spasmodic dysphonia. *Journal of Laryngology and Otology* 119 (3), 222–225.

Tsuzuki, T., Fukuda, H., Fujioka, T., Takayama, E. and Kawaida, M. (1991) Voice prognosis after liquid and solid silicone injection. *American Journal of Otolaryngology* 12 (3), 165–169.

Tucker, H. (1976) Human laryngeal reinnervation. *Laryngoscope* 86 (6), 769–779.

Von Leden, H. (1971) Phonosurgery. *Acta Oto-Rino-Laringológica Ibero-Americana* 22 (3), 291–299.

Yamaguchi, H., Yotsukura, Y., Sata, H., Watanabe, Y., Hirose, H., Kobayashi, N., *et al.* (1993) Pushing exercise program to correct glottal incompetence. *Journal of Voice* 7 (3), 250–256.

Yumoto, E., Sanuki, T., Toya, Y., Kodama, N. and Kumai, Y. (2010) Nerve-muscle pedicle flap implantation combined with arytenoid adduction. *Archives of Otolaryngology – Head and Neck Surgery* 136 (10), 965–969.

# 8   Current Issues in Voice Assessment and Intervention in the United Kingdom

## Paul Carding

## The UK National Health Service and Voice Disorders

Services for voice disordered patients in the United Kingdom are delivered within the context of the National Health Service (NHS).[1] The NHS is the world's largest publicly funded health service. It is also one of the most efficient, most egalitarian and most comprehensive.The founding principle is that high quality healthcare should be available to all, regardless of wealth. The NHS remains free at the point of use for anyone who is resident in the UK. The money to pay for the NHS comes directly from national taxation. According to independent bodies such as the King's Fund, this remains the 'cheapest and fairest' way of funding health care when compared with other systems. The 2008–2009 budget roughly equates to a contribution of £1980 for every man, woman and child in the UK.

The NHS employs more than 1.7 million people and has a budget of more than £100 billion. According to national statistics it deals with 1 million patients every 36 hours. That's 463 people a minute or almost eight a second! Each week, 700,000 people will visit an NHS dentist, while a further 3000 will have a heart operation. It is estimated that there are at least 50,000 new cases of dysphonia every year in the UK (Carding, 2003a).

The NHS is divided into two sections: primary and secondary care. Primary care is the first point of contact for most people and is delivered by a wide range of independent contractors, including general practitioners, dentists and pharmacists.Therefore, most people who have a voice problem would go to their general practitioner in the first instance. Secondary care is also known as acute healthcare or hospital healthcare. This is where specialist medical or paramedical healthcare happens. Access to secondary healthcare services is usually through referral from a primary or community health professional such as a general practitioner. Secondary care clinicians can refer to each other within the acute hospitals without any concerns about payment. Some acute hospitals are regional or national centres for more specialised care. They may be attached to universities and help to train health professionals. The great majority of services for voice disordered patients are conducted in the acute/hospital setting for obvious reasons.

The NHS also oversees the National Institute for Health and Clinical Excellence (NICE). NICE is the independent organisation responsible for providing national guidance on the promotion of good health and the prevention and treatment of ill health. NICE also produces evidence-based guidance on aspects such as health technologies (guidance on the use of new and existing medicines, treatments and procedures) and clinical practice (guidance on the appropriate treatment and care of people with specific diseases and conditions).

NICE makes recommendations to the NHS on (a) new and existing medicines, treatments and procedures (e.g. percutaneous injections for vocal fold paralysis) and (b) treating and caring for people with specific diseases and conditions (e.g. surgical treatment of spasmodic dysphonia). NICE also runs a Google-style database called NHS Evidence. This allows NHS staff to search the internet for up-to-date evidence of effectiveness and examples of best practice in relation to health and social care. NICE is also developing and defining the standards of healthcare that people can expect to receive. These standards will indicate when a clinical treatment (or set of clinical procedures) is considered highly effective, cost effective and safe, as well as being viewed as a positive experience by patients. It is anticipated that these standards will be agreed for many areas of voice pathology within the next few years.

This national framework and funding for voice disorder services has both advantages and disadvantages. The services are funded throughout the country and can be accessed free by all patients. This may be compared to, for example, France, where estimates are that approximately 80% of voice provision is provided by the independent, that is non-government funded, sector. The NHS arrangement does, however, produce some interesting issues and debates. For example, are all voice problems health-related problems (e.g. singing difficulties) or how long should a course of treatment last and what criteria for discharge should be employed? Because there are no insurance or personal payment issues, the treating clinician is free to design a programme of therapy that is specific to the individual and (if appropriate) be eclectic in the type of therapy offered. This requires highly skilled clinicians who are trained in a comprehensive range of treatment approaches and who have sufficient experience of when to apply what technique and when to change approach (if necessary).

## Voice Services in the UK

In recent years, the UK has seen a considerable increase in clinical and research resources for voice disorders. This expansion is largely due to additional governmental funding for head and neck cancer services and the general expansion of voice clinic services (Carding, 2003a). Almost every city has a designated specialist voice clinic, which is a joint consultation clinic involving both a laryngologist and an expert speech/voice pathology clinician – often called 'voice therapists' (Figure 8.1). These traditional voice clinics are equipped with a full range of endoscopic and stroboscopic diagnostic equipment. The core personnel would always include a laryngologist and an expert speech and language therapist (specialising in voice disorders). These clinicians would be expected to offer a comprehensive range of medical, phonosurgical, logaoedic and behavioural treatments.

However, not all centres would attempt to offer all highly specialised services for relatively uncommon disorders (e.g. botulinum toxin injections for spasmodic dysphonia or cognitive–behavioural therapy for some types of functional dysphonia). In these cases, the transfer of patients to colleagues elsewhere in the region/country is easily facilitated. Some voice clinics have additional expert personnel such as singing teachers, clinical psychologists

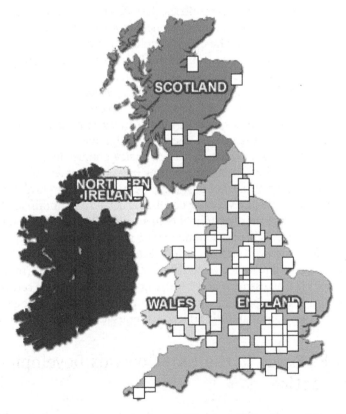

**Figure 8.1** A schematic representation of UK voice clinics (as registered with the British Voice Association, 2009)

and/or osteopaths. However, these are not common and are usually only available in the private sector and not as part of the National Health Service.

Only in the very largest conurbations would competing clinical facilities exist and hence there is (generally) little benefit in the advertising and promotion of individual centres. All of these clinics are provided within the National Health Service (NHS) and are free to all UK citizens. Due to the population density of the UK, this situation means that most patients are relatively near to a specialist voice centre. In rural areas, a 'hub and spoke' model has usually been established – where 'satellite clinics' refer into the central areas of excellence whenever necessary. Despite the common political debate in the UK about the relative merits of providing 'localised health service delivery' (as opposed to centralised/super-hospital based delivery), this hub and spoke model is unlikely to change for a condition as specialised as voice disorders.

## Expert Practitioner Roles in the UK

Unlike most other European countries, the UK does not have a phoniatrician-based voice service. All medical practitioners involved in voice disorders services are surgically trained. The otolaryngological sub-speciality within the Royal College of Surgeons has often debated specialist training in phoniatric skills but no formalised syllabus has yet emerged.

The voice/speech pathologist's role and the services that these clinicians provide in UK voice practice are developing rapidly (e.g. Carding, 2003a, 2003b). In many cases this has meant a change in the relationship between the laryngologist and voice pathologist/therapist and a development of the range of voice services that are available. All university courses in speech and language therapy will include intensive teaching in voice disorders and their management. A significant number of postgraduate specialist courses also exist and it is incumbent upon the individual specialist clinician to maintain and develop their postgraduate training portfolio. Frequent initiatives to 'modernise' NHS service delivery have resulted in extended roles for voice/speech pathologists in the UK (see, for example, Carding, 2003b; Rattenbury et al., 2004). For example, it is now commonplace for voice/speech pathologists to perform laryngeal endoscopy for both assessment and treatment purposes. In some centres is not uncommon for highly specialist voice/speech pathologists to be the first consultation point for some carefully triaged patient groups (Carding, 2003b).

## Clinical Research in the UK – Towards Developing Better Practice

The great majority of UK voice research is done by practising clinicians and, subsequently, most of the topics are of direct clinical value. We believe that this arrangement is crucial for the future of the speciality. The principles of evidence-based practice are firmly established in the national clinical guidelines for voice/speech pathologists (Taylor-Goh, 2004). It is acknowledged that highly specialised clinical practice and clinical research are necessary (and inevitable) partners. Specialist clinicians are expected to generate clinical questions and to seek the means to answer them (i.e. via good quality research).

For all of these reasons it is not surprising that one main area of UK research productivity relates to treatment efficacy/effectiveness and its corollary – treatment outcome measurement (Carding, 2000). UK publications on speech and language treatment (generally) have grown by over 50% in the past 15 years. The UK is the second most productive country in research output, publishing 12% of the world's publication output (Lewison & Carding, 2003). Voice research is one area of increasing strength. According to Robey's five-phase model of clinical outcome research (Robey, 2004), voice research has confidently entered into phases 3 (large-scale efficacy studies) and 4 (effectiveness studies). Pring (2004) suggests that this may be because the field of voice disorders enjoys (relative to many other areas of speech and language pathology) clear(er) diagnostic categories, better agreement on treatment aims and more defined treatment outcome measures.

The UK has provided some seminal treatment efficacy studies in non-organic voice disorders. These include one of the first major prospective group studies (Carding et al., 1999) and the first randomised controlled trial (MacKenzie et al., 2001). Partly due to these studies, the treatment of non-organic dysphonia (the most common type of voice disorder) is considered efficacious. Other significant UK treatment effectiveness studies have followed (e.g. Gillivan-Murphy et al., 2006; Rattenbury et al., 2004).

As a natural corollary to this clinical focus of our research activity, a number of UK publications have followed in the refinement and usage of voice outcome measures. These include publications about new patient-report instruments (Deary et al., 2003), patient self-ratings of voice quality (Lee et al., 2005) and the design of voice assessment material (Abberton, 2005). Perhaps more importantly, UK voice clinicians have contributed important studies examining the reliability, validity and sensitivity to change, and utility of existing voice measures (Carding et al., 2004; Deary et al., 2004; Steen et al., 2008; Webb et al., 2004, 2007; Wilson et al., 2004). A review of these (and other key) studies was published in 2009 (Carding et al., 2009).

With continued close liaison between clinical and research activity, voice/speech pathologists are well placed to further contribute to the evidence base of voice disorders and their treatment. The juxtaposition of clinical and research skills means that further studies of treatment effectiveness (rather than efficacy) are certainly possible and desirable. These ventures are likely to involve multicentre (and multi-clinician) studies. These methodological designs will enable the analysis of otherwise uncommon disorders and examine the effectiveness of voice therapy *practice* (i.e. treatment pro-grammes conducted by different clinicians) rather than the effectiveness of an individual voice therapist. There are also indications that the psychological aspects of voice disorders require considerable research attention. Previous efficacy studies have suggested that psychological features do not improve following traditional voice therapy (e.g. MacKenzie *et al.*, 2001). A question remains as to whether voice therapy should reasonably aim to change these aspects of the patient and, if so, how (this subject is addressed further in another chapter in this book).

## Notes

(1)  There is a private sector for health care in the UK. This represents no more than 2% of healthcare provision in the UK and is most frequently used for elective procedures.

## References

Abberton, D.E. (2005) Phonetic considerations in the design of voice assessment material. *Logopedics Phonatrics Vocology* 30 (3–4), 175–180.

Carding, P.N. (2000) *Measuring the Effectiveness of Treatment*. London: Whurr Publishers. ISBN 1 86156 162 8.

Carding, P.N. (2003a) Voice pathology in the United Kingdom. *British Medical Journal* 327 (7414), 514–515.

Carding, P.N. (2003b) Voice pathology clinics in the UK. *Clinical Otolaryngology & Allied Sciences* 28 (6), 477–478.

Carding, P.N., Horsley, I.A. and Docherty, G.J. (1999) A study of the effectiveness of voice therapy in the treatment of 45 patients with nonorganic dysphonia. *Journal of Voice* 13 (1), 72–104.

Carding, P., Steen, I., Webb, A., Mackenzie, K., Deary, I. and Wilson, J. (2004) The reliability and sensitivity to change of acoustic measures of voice quality. *Clinical Otolaryngology & Allied Sciences* 29 (5), 538–544.

Carding, P.N., Wilson, J.A., MacKenzie, K. and Deary, I.J. (2009) Measuring voice outcomes: A state of the science review. *Journal of Laryngology and Otology* 123 (8), 823–829.

Deary, I., Wilson, J., Carding, P. and MacKenzie, K. (2003) VoiSS: A patient-derived Voice Symptom Scale. *Journal of Psychosomatic Research* 54 (5), 483–489.

Deary, I., Webb, A., MacKenzie, K., Wilson, J. and Carding, P. (2004) Short, self-report voice symptom scales: Psychometric characteristics of the Voice Handicap Index-10 and the Vocal Performance Questionnaire. *Head & Neck Surgery* 131, 232–235.

Gillivan-Murphy, P., Drinnan, M., O'Dwyer, T., Ridha, H. and Carding, P. (2006) The effectiveness of a voice treatment approach for teachers with self-reported voice problems. *Journal of Voice* 20 (3), 423–431.

Lee, M., Drinnan, M. and Carding, P. (2005) The reliability and validity of patient self rating of their own voice quality. *Clinical Otolaryngology* 30 (4), 357–361.

Lewison, G. and Carding, P. (2003) Evaluating UK research in speech and language therapy. *International Journal of Language & Communication Disorders* 38 (1), 65–84.

MacKenzie, K., Millar, A., Wilson, J., Sellars, C. and Deary, I. (2001) Is voice therapy an effective treatment for dysphonia? A randomised controlled trial. *British Medical Journal* 323 (7314), 658–661.

Pring, T. (2004) Ask a silly question: Two decades of troublesome trials. *International Journal of Language & Communication Disorders* 39 (3), 285–302.

Rattenbury, H., Carding, P. and Finn, P. (2004) Evaluating the effectiveness and efficiency of voice therapy using transnasal flexible laryngoscopy: A randomized controlled trial. *Journal of Voice* 18 (4), 522–533.

Robey, R. (2004) A five-phase model for clinical-outcome research. *Journal of Communication Disorders* 37 (5), 401–411.

Steen, I., MacKenzie, K., Carding, P., Webb, A., Deary, I. and Wilson, J. (2008) Optimising outcome assessment of voice interventions. II: Sensitivity to change of self-reported and observer-rated measures. *Journal of Laryngology and Otology* 122 (1), 46–51.

Taylor-Goh, S. (ed.) (2004) *Evidence Based Clinical Guidelines*. London: Royal College of Speech and Language Therapists.

Webb, A., Carding, P., Deary, I., MacKenzie, K., Steen, N. and Wilson, J. (2004) The reliability of three perceptual evaluation scales for dysphonia. *European Archives of Oto-Rhino-Laryngology* 261 (8), 429–434.

Webb, A., Carding, P., Deary, I., MacKenzie, K., Steen, I. and Wilson, J. (2007) Optimising outcome assessment of voice interventions. I: Reliability and validity of three self-reported scales. *Journal of Laryngology and Otology* 121 (8), 763–767.

Wilson, J., Webb, A., Carding, P., Steen, I., MacKenzie, K. and Deary, I. (2004) The Voice Symptom Scale (VoiSS) and the Vocal Handicap Index (VHI): A comparison of structure and content. *Clinical Otolaryngology & Allied Sciences* 29 (2), 169–174.

# 9 Current Issues in Voice Assessment and Intervention in the USA

## Tanya L. Eadie and Edie R. Hapner

In the United States of America (USA), it is estimated that 3–10% of the population experience voice problems at any one moment in time, with approximately one-third of all Americans reporting impaired voice production at some point in their lives (Roy *et al.*, 2004). While there is a relatively high incidence of voice disorders in the USA, only 5.9% of those in the general population who experience dysphonia reportedly seek treatment. The relative lack of awareness about voice disorders and their underlying causes among the general population and health professionals have been cited as potential barriers to appropriate care (Schwartz *et al.*, 2009). In contrast to many other countries, inadequate insurance coverage may also be a cause of failure to seek treatment for dysphonia in the USA, and may even result in delayed diagnosis and treatment of life-threatening diseases (Chen *et al.*, 2007).

The diagnosis, assessment, treatment and prevention of voice disorders fall under the purview of a number of disciplines, including otolaryngology–head and neck surgery, speech-language pathology, neurology, professional voice and singing teaching, family medicine, pulmonology, geriatric medicine, nursing, internal medicine, psychiatry and pediatrics. However, physicians are the only professionals qualified and licensed to render medical diagnoses related to the identification of laryngeal pathology as it affects voice (ASHA, 1998). Ideally, medical diagnoses related to laryngeal pathologies are made by (oto)laryngologists who have developed expertise in this area through the completion of a one-year fellowship in laryngology, following complete ear-nose-throat training. Laryngology training, therefore, is akin to 'phoniatrics training' in many European countries (Rubin *et al.*, 2007).

Certified and licensed speech-language pathologists are the health care professionals in the USA who have the expertise to provide functional assessment and effective behavioral treatment for dysphonia (ASHA, 2004b, 2005c). Speech-language pathologists are governed by the American Speech-Language-Hearing Association (ASHA), as well as the laws of the individual state in which the clinician practices. According to ASHA, speech-language patholo-gists hold the ASHA Certificate of Clinical Competence in Speech-Language Pathology (CCC-SLP), which requires a master's, doctoral or other recognized post-baccalaureate degree. Speech-language pathologists provide prevention, screening, consultation, assessment, treatment, intervention, management, counseling and follow-up services for individuals with communication and swallowing disorders (ASHA, 2004b, 2007). The framework used to provide assessment and treatment is consistent with the World Health Organization (WHO)'s *International Classification of Functioning, Disability and Health* (WHO, 2001). As such, clinical voice practice involves a broad range of services, from assessing the function of the vocal folds via laryngovideostroboscopy, to facil-itating performance of a work presentation, to providing counseling about total laryngectomy (Ma *et al.*, 2007).

To ensure competent and ethical services, speech-language pathologists who provide services to individuals with voice disorders may require special-ized training and knowledge above and beyond CCC-SLP certification, par-ticularly in the areas of vocal tract visualization and imaging, instrumentation and selection/placement of tracheoesophageal prostheses (ASHA, 2004a, 2004b). To promote professional interests, develop policy and ensure contin-ued education, speech-language pathologists also may become members of ASHA Special Interest Group 3, Voice and Voice Disorders – one of 18 ASHA Special Interest Groups (http://www.asha.org/SIG/). Special Interest Group 3 includes approximately 1700 members (i.e. representing fewer than 10% of the Special Interest Group membership). This small percentage is representa-tive of the proportion of speech-language pathologists who provide services to those with dysphonia, with membership represented across a number of service models, including private practitioners, members of hospital-based speech-language pathology departments, members of an otolaryngology or other medical specialty department, members of a skilled nursing facility, or school-based clinicians, to name a few.

The purpose of this chapter is to address specific issues in clinical voice assessment and intervention related to practice in the USA. The gold stan-dard approach to assessment and treatment of dysphonia is supported by an interdisciplinary approach, as reflected in documents from ASHA, the American Academy of Otolaryngology–Head and Neck Surgery (AAO-HNS), the National Association of Teachers of Singing (NATS), and the Voice and Speech Trainers Association (VASTA) (ASHA, 1998, 2005b; Schwartz *et al.*, 2009). However, there are a number of challenges to implementation that are related to the cultural, social and economic milieu within practice settings. While patients and clinicians alike benefit from an interdisciplinary team approach, it is important to recognize that, in some clinical practice settings, professionals (e.g. speech-language pathologists, otolaryngologists) may not always be located in one facility. As a result, it is critical to build relationships within the community to maximize patient care. Access to resources also varies from setting to setting, as do service delivery models and clinical populations served. The diverse linguistic and cultural background of each patient also challenges the clinician to find appropriate and valid assessment tools and treatment methods (ASHA, 2004b; DeJarnette & Holland, 1998). Finally, there is always the balance between an evidence-based approach to assessment and treatment and the need to streamline due to time constraints and insurance reimbursement. These forces can often influence the timing of assessments, as well as how many therapy sessions (if at all) are reimbursed, which may become ethical dilemmas for speech-language pathologists. These challenges are highlighted in the following sections related to voice assessment and treatment in the USA.

## Issues Related to Voice Assessment in the USA

Recently, the AAO-HNS established clinical practice guidelines for treating hoarseness (dysphonia), based on recommendations from an interdisciplinary panel (Schwartz et al., 2009). First, the panel recommended that physicians diagnose dysphonia in patients with altered voice quality, pitch, loudness or vocal effort that impairs communication or reduces voice-related quality of life. The purpose of this recommendation was to recognize dysphonia as a symptom that may need further investigation to determine underlying conditions, and to discourage the perception of dysphonia (hoarseness) as trivial. It also was recommended that physicians assess a patient with hoarseness by history and/or physical examination, with particular attention focused on factors that might modify management, such as recent surgical procedures involving the neck, endotracheal intubation, radiation treatment, history of tobacco and alcohol use, and occupation as a singer or vocal performer (Schwartz et al., 2009). Finally, it was recommended that physicians visualize the patient's larynx, or refer the patient to a clinician who could visual the larynx (via laryngoscopy), when hoarseness fails to resolve by a maximum of three months after onset (or irrespective of duration if a serious underlying cause is suspected). Thus, at a minimum, when a patient with dysphonia is evaluated, the basic protocol should include a rigorous clinical history, performance of a physical examination, and visualization of the larynx via laryngoscopy.

The gold standard clinical care for patients with dysphonia in the USA involves a team approach between an otolaryngologist and a speech-language pathologist with expertise in voice care (Benninger et al., 1994). The assumption is that the combination of both disciplines results in better treatment than by either discipline in isolation. In some settings, voice evaluations are performed simultaneously by the otolaryngologist and speech-language pathologist. However, even within interdisciplinary settings, there is wide variability related to whether the entire evaluation is performed as a team or whether one team member performs a preliminary evaluation before being reviewed by the second team member. In addition, some settings are not conducive to joint evaluations (e.g. school-based, private practice), which alters the nature of the communication between team members.

While these evaluations may be performed separately, one important caveat is that a speech-language pathologist must *not initiate treatment* until a medical diagnosis is provided and there is expected benefit from behavioral intervention (ASHA, 2004b; Schwartz *et al.*, 2009). In addition, while some of the instruments/tools used during the evaluation (e.g. laryngovideostroboscopy, case history or quality of life measurement) may be similar between otolaryngologists and speech-language pathologists, the purpose of the evaluation is different for each team member. The physician's objective is to render medical diagnoses related to the identification of laryngeal pathology and to determine appropriate management strategies (e.g. referral for voice therapy via a certified speech-language pathologist, watchful waiting, steroids, surgery, anti-reflux medication) (Schwartz *et al.*, 2009). Before rendering a diagnosis, the physician may need information from other professionals (e.g. pulmonologists, neurologists, gastroenterologists), and results from other tests (e.g. diagnostic imaging procedures). The objective of the speech-language pathology evaluation is to assess voice production and function and to determine how the voice disorder affects an individual in everyday communication contexts, as well as to determine prognosis for change, provide recommendations for intervention and support, and to recommend referrals where appropriate (ASHA, 1998, 2004b).

In contrast with the European Laryngological Society (ELS), there is not one standardized protocol recommended for the functional assessment of voice pathology in the USA (Dejonckere *et al.*, 2001). While practice guidelines by both ASHA and the AAO-HNS recommend general approaches to assessment, there remains wide variability in which voice measures are used to determine vocal pathology and diagnosis of the severity of dysphonia (ASHA, 2004b; Schwartz *et al.*, 2009). This variability creates difficulties across centers because measures and terminology may remain somewhat inconsistent, making it difficult to compare clinical outcomes and interpret results. A standard, albeit not necessarily typical, approach is described below.

Despite variability between settings, most clinics have developed standardized clinical intake forms, which direct further questions during a clinical history interview about relevant medical, behavioral and psychosocial history, as well as voice use/demands, voice training history, vocal hygiene practices and the patient's chief complaints. The history also allows time to develop rapport, and to take into account any unique history or vocal demands that may differentiate either the specific diagnosis or the severity of the voice problem.

After a comprehensive voice history is performed, self-report measures are used to supplement the history and document other symptoms (e.g. laryngopharyngeal reflux via the Reflux Symptom Index (RSI); Belafsky *et al.*, 2002). Other self-report measures (e.g. the Voice Handicap Index; Jacobson *et al.*, 1997) are used to quantitatively measure the impact of the voice disorder on a person's everyday life. Patients also are often asked to self-evaluate their voice quality and effort. Information derived from self-report instruments helps determine the etiology of the voice problem (e.g. RSI), and may be used for therapy outcomes assessment. It should be noted that interpretation of results must be performed in light of the linguistic and cultural background of the patient, age and other demographic factors, as well as vocational and voice demands (ASHA, 2004b). In practice, self-report tools are often completed prior to visiting a speech-language pathologist or otolaryngologist, and are then discussed during the case history. This approach helps streamline evaluation time.

Following the case history and the patient's perception of the problem, a head and neck examination and a detailed laryngeal examination are performed by the physician. The purpose of the head and neck examination is to rule out any malignancy causing the dysphonia, and to determine any co-morbid medical conditions that might affect the voice (e.g. sinus allergies, laryngopharyngeal reflux). A laryngeal examination is then performed using laryngoscopy. The type of examination (transorally using a mirror or transnasally with a flexible fiber optic laryngoscope) depends on the preference/expertise of the physician performing the examination, the patient's tolerance of the procedure, the specific (or suspected) diagnoses, and the resources/equipment available in the center. Unfortunately, there are no guidelines for physicians regarding which type of visualization procedure to use when making a diagnosis. Thus, some physicians in the USA still diagnose laryngeal pathologies based on mirror exams and refer for voice therapy. Other physicians will then refer for videostroboscopy if it is not available in their clinics. The gold standard in specialized voice clinics remains laryngovideostroboscopy using either flexible or rigid endoscopes (Sataloff *et al.*, 1991).

Laryngovideostroboscopy is sometimes performed by speech-language pathologists in conjunction with (or in addition to) otolaryngologists to determine vocal function, to use as an educational tool or to use as therapeutic biofeedback (Behrman, 2005). The use of this tool requires specialized training, and equipment is not typically found beyond specialized interdisciplinary voice centers (ASHA, 2004a). The use of laryngovideostroboscopy by speech-language pathologists has another caveat. Insurance companies have changed the extent of physician oversight required multiple times over the past several years. While ASHA and the AAO-HNS agree that speech-language pathologists are among the medical professionals skilled in performing laryngovideostroboscopy, individual states mandate the scope of practice guidelines (ASHA, 2007; Schwartz *et al.*, 2009).

Speech-language pathologists may perform a number of evaluations that document baseline vocal functioning, and help determine a functional voice diagnosis. These measures also provide values that may be used as therapeutic outcome measures. The current standard for auditory-perceptual evaluation of dysphonia includes the Consensus Auditory-Perceptual Evaluation of Voice (CAPE-V) (ASHA, 2002; Kempster et al., 2009), which involves the judgment of a number of voice parameters using 100 mm visual analog scales. In a survey of experienced voice clinicians (all speech-language pathologists), Behrman (2005) found that 100% of the respondents used auditory-perceptual measures during voice evaluation. However, it remains unclear how many speech-language pathologists continue to use their own scales and definitions of voice qualities when yielding these responses, which reduces the reliability of these measures (Kreiman et al., 1993). A standardized approach such as the CAPE-V will address some sources of variability, with a potential future for anchor samples and training that could promote inter-rater reliability (Kempster et al., 2009). These approaches are already advocated in other countries (e.g. ELS protocol, Japan, Australia), but vary in terms of the scale types and definitions used for dysphonic qualities (Dejonckere et al., 2001; Hirano, 1981; Oates & Russell, 1998).

In addition to auditory-perceptual measures, various objective measures (e.g. acoustics, aerodynamic, electroglottographic) are often performed by speech-language pathologists. Behrman (2005) noted that voice quality, observation of body posture and movement and probing the patient's ability to alter voice production were significantly more likely to be assessed during evaluations than stroboscopic, acoustic, aerodynamic and electroglottographic measures. The challenges to performing instrumental measures include limited resources and expertise for using equipment, as well as time constraints for performing evaluations. It is clear that further training is necessary in this area to ensure the validity of these measures for a variety of patient populations (DeJarnette & Holland, 1998). Many of these issues related to assessment also pertain to constraints on how speech-language pathologists perform voice therapy and are addressed in the following sections.

## Issues Related to Voice Therapy in the USA

Voice therapy in the USA works within a fee for service system. The costs of voice therapy have traditionally been covered by insurance companies and by Medicare, the government controlled medical health system of payment for people over 65 years (Centers for Medicare and Medicaid Services, 2008). Changes in the healthcare system have resulted in reductions in insurance reimbursements for voice therapy, and have forced speech-language pathologists to streamline therapeutic efforts (e.g. a typical regimen of reimbursed voice therapy includes six face-to-face sessions). In a recent article, insurance reimbursement was one of the most frequently occurring reasons for people to refuse voice therapy or stop attending (Hapner et al.,

2009). New service delivery models have emerged in response to the need to 'get it done faster with less face time'. Telehealth (Brown *et al.*, 2010), use of virtual therapists (Cole *et al.*, 2006) and methods to increase adherence to home programs (van Leer & Connor, 2010) to lessen face-to-face contact time have developed in response to less insurance coverage for voice therapy.

With these issues in mind, current approaches to voice therapy in the USA have vastly changed since their inception. One method that has remained a staple of voice therapy includes hygienic voice therapy (Thomas & Stemple, 2007). The general philosophy underlying this method is that some vocal behaviors cause trauma to the delicate laryngeal structures and that eliminating those behaviors will improve vocal performance. Approaches include educating the patient about the vocal mechanism, reducing phonotraumatic behaviors (e.g. yelling, throat-clearing), managing co-morbidities that increase risk of damage to the vocal folds (or have already caused damage, such as laryngopharyngeal reflux) and promoting behaviors that may facilitate healing and reduce vocal load (e.g. hydration, using amplification).

In general, hygienic voice therapy is not used alone but rather as a part of a comprehensive voice therapy program (Behrman *et al.*, 2008; Thomas & Stemple, 2007). For example, vocal hygiene typically is addressed and monitored throughout voice therapy, with time constraints in therapeutic face-to-face contact time limiting more comprehensive coverage. Recent research comparing vocal hygiene (education, hydration) and more direct voice therapy methods has indicated that voice hygiene alone is not as effective in improving voice quality as more direct therapeutic regimes (Behrman *et al.*, 2008; Roy *et al.*, 2002, 2003). The one exception to this rule is the use of voice amplification, which alone has shown positive outcomes (on par with some direct therapy approaches) in teachers (Roy *et al.*, 2002).

In addition to vocal hygiene approaches, most speech-language pathologists in the USA use some form of direct voice therapy (i.e. symptomatic and physiologic therapies) for treating individuals with voice disorders. Symptomatic voice therapy methods, introduced in the early 1970s by Dr Daniel Boone, have undergone a number of changes over the years (Boone *et al.*, 2005). Symptomatic therapy addresses the respiratory, phonatory, resonatory, articulatory and postural presentation of the person with dysphonia (Boone, 1971). The method suggests that, by modifying the symptom to a more normal voice quality, the voice problem will improve. For example, if the pitch of the voice is too high, the suggestion is to lower the pitch to one that is normal for the person's age, gender and stature. There are also a few techniques (called facilitators) whose goal is to address inappropriate loudness, as well as excessive jaw or vocal tension such as a yawn-sigh or chewing.

Several symptomatic techniques continue to be used today, such as chant talk, glottal fry and tongue protrusion (Behrman *et al.*, 2008). However, several techniques have fallen out of favor, including pushing to increase glottal closure, as well as establishing optimal pitch (Branski *et al.*, 2008). In general, efficacy studies have failed to demonstrate that any particular facilitating technique is useful in the remediation of dysphonia. Rather, studies have examined the use of several techniques simultaneously, with findings that the symptomatic approach as a whole is useful (Thomas & Stemple, 2007).

An increasingly used approach in voice therapy includes etiologic (so-called physiologic) approaches. Physiologic voice therapy techniques balance the three subsystems of voice production: respiration, phonation and resonance, with the restoration of balance resulting in increased vocal efficiency (Stemple & Fry, 2010). While one of the first physiologic treatment protocols, the Accent Method (Kotby *et al.*, 1981), was developed in Egypt, many physiologic voice therapy methods have their origins in the USA, including: Lessac–Madsen Resonant Voice Therapy (Verdolini, 1998), Vocal Function Exercises (Stemple *et al.*, 1994), and Lee Silverman Voice Treatment (Ramig *et al.*, 2004). In general, these approaches have the highest levels of therapeutic evidence (Thomas & Stemple, 2007).

A final method used in voice therapy includes a psychogenic approach. In the 1980s, Arnold Aronson reintroduced the concept that some dysphonia may be related to problems with overall emotional stability manifested in the voice. Psychogenic voice therapy was aimed at 'releasing the inherently normal voice suppressed by excessive muscular tension' (Aronson, 1980: 195). Aronson (1980) noted that this release could be accomplished through mechanically relaxing the musculature or by psychologically releasing the anxiety causing the tension. He described a physical manipulation of the larynx, called laryngeal massage, to mechanically lower the larynx in the throat. This general approach has continued to be modified by others, with demonstrated positive outcomes (Roy & Leeper, 1993).

To be proficient in using the psychogenic voice therapy paradigm, clinicians are expected to perform a significant amount of patient counseling and have a ready armament of skilled psychologists to participate in therapy when needed. To date, training graduate-level students to become speech-language pathologists in the USA requires no specific coursework in counseling beyond a demonstration of basic skills in clinical practice or coursework (ASHA, 2005a). However, the use of counseling approaches, such as motivational interviewing, may increase adherence to voice therapy, resulting in improved outcomes (Behrman, 2006; van Leer & Connor, 2010). The ability to develop expertise in these areas and to incorporate these strategies into limited therapeutic time remains a challenge for voice clinicians.

# Implications for Future Clinical Practice

While the percentage of ASHA members interested in voice is small, the Voice and Voice Disorders Special Interest Group 3 posted its largest membership

in early 2011, reflecting an increased interest among speech-language pathologists in the area of voice care. Yet in a survey of affiliates of ASHA's Group 3
(previously called Division 3) completed in 2006, the majority of the membership reported that less than 25% of their caseload is the evaluation and treatment of voice disorders. The low numbers of speech-language pathologists
working in the area of voice in the USA has hindered support from ASHA-
based research initiatives. Speech-language pathologists also find themselves
frequently having to justify services, especially in the voice arena, to insurance payers. This seeming tug of war between using diagnostically sensitive
assessment tools, efficacious voice therapy, recommendations by the AAO-
HNS to use voice therapy in the treatment of dysphonia, and the yearly reduction of fees paid by insurance companies for voice therapy has frustrated many
voice therapists.

However, the mandated use of an evidence-based approach has resulted in
a rapid increase in knowledge about voice disorders, as well as their assessment
and treatment. A new generation of voice disorders research has emerged to
complement the physiologically based paradigms used in evaluation and treatment. Speech scientists and clinicians have begun to work in tandem from
bench research through clinical practice (Branski & Lodewyck, 2006). Translational research in the USA is forcing speech-language pathologists to learn
rudimentary information on vocal fold tissue dynamics, air flows and pres-
sures, and histology, while equally forcing researchers to consider the application of their findings to patient care. No longer is expert opinion acceptable
when discussing the use of assessment or therapy techniques. Rather, evidence-
based practice has become the expected norm. By accepting these challenges,
the care of those with voice disorders within the USA continues to improve.

# References

Aronson, A. (1980) *Clinical Voice Disorders: An Interdisciplinary Approach.* New York: Brian
    C. Decker.
ASHA (1998) The roles of otolaryngologists and speech-language pathologists in the per-
    formance and interpretation of strobovideolaryngoloscopy. Relevant paper, accessed
    8 July 2010. http://www.asha.org/docs/html/RP1998-00132.html
ASHA (2002) *Consensus Auditory-Perceptual Evaluation of Voice (CAPE-V).* Rockville Pike:
    American-Speech-Language-Hearing Association.
ASHA (2004a) Knowledge and skills for speech-language pathologists with respect to
    vocal tract visualization and imaging. *ASHA Supplement* 24, 184–192.
ASHA (2004b) Preferred practice patterns for the profession of speech-language pathol-
    ogy. Preferred practice pattern, accessed 11 July 2010. http://www.asha.org/docs/
    html/PP2004-00191.html
ASHA (2005a) Frequently asked questions about the 2005 Certification Standards in
    Speech-Language Pathology, accessed 11 July 2010. http://www.asha.org/certifica
    tion/2005_SLP_FAQ.htm
ASHA (2005b) The role of the speech-language pathologist, the teacher of singing, and
    the speaking voice training in voice habilitation. Technical report, accessed 11 July
    2010. http://www.asha.org/docs/html/TR2005-00147.html

ASHA (2005c) The use of voice therapy in the treatment of dysphonia. Technical report, accessed 11 July 2010. http://www.asha.org/docs/html/TR2005-00158.html

ASHA (2007) Scope of practice in speech-language pathology. Scope of practice, accessed 11 July 2010. http://www.asha.org/policy/SP2007-00283/

Behrman, A. (2005) Common practices of voice therapists in the evaluation of patients. *Journal of Voice* 19 (3), 454–469.

Behrman, A. (2006) Facilitating behavioral change in voice therapy: The relevance of motivational interviewing. *American Journal of Speech-Language Pathology* 15, 215–225.

Behrman, A., Rutledge, J., Hembree, A. and Sheridan, S. (2008) Voice hygiene education, voice production therapy, and the role of patient adherence: A treatment effectiveness study in women with phonotrauma. *Journal of Speech, Language, and Hearing Research* 51 (2), 350–366.

Belafsky, P.C., Postma, G.N. and Koufman, J.A. (2002) Validity and reliability of the reflux symptom index (RSI). *Journal of Voice* 16 (2), 274–277.

Benninger, M.S., Jacobson, B.H. and Johnson, A. (1994) *Vocal Arts Medicine: The Care and Prevention of Professional Voice Disorders*. New York: Thieme Medical Publishers.

Boone, D. (1971) *The Voice and Voice Therapy*. New Jersey: Prentice-Hall.

Boone, D., McFarlane, S. and Von Berg, S. (2005) *The Voice and Voice Therapy* (8th edn). Boston: Allyn & Bacon.

Branski, R.C. and Lodewyck, D.N. (2006) Emerging basic science and voice disorders. Article, accessed 10 July 2010. http://www.speechpathology.com/articles/article_detail.asp?article_id=300

Branski, R., Murry, T. and Rosen, C. (2008) Voice therapy. Article, accessed 11 July 2010. http://emedicine.medscape.com/article/866712-overview

Brown, J., Brannon, J. and Romanow, K. (2010) Reimbursement for telespeech. *Perspectives on Voice and Voice Disorders* 20, 16–21.

Centers for Medicare and Medicaid Services (2008) *What is Medicare?* Accessed 10 July 2010. http://www.medicare.gov/Publications/Pubs/pdf/11306.pdf

Chen, A.Y., Schrag, N.M., Halpern, M., Stewart, A. and Ward, E.M. (2007) Health insurance and stage at diagnosis of laryngeal cancer. *Archives of Otolaryngology – Head & Neck Surgery* 133 (8), 784–790.

Cole, R., Halpern, A., Ramig, L., Vuuren, S., Ngampatipatpong, N. and Yan, J. (2006) A virtual speech therapist for individuals with Parkinson's disease. *Educational Technology* 47 (1), 51–55.

DeJarnette, G. and Holland, R.W. (1998) Voice and voice disorders. In D.E. Battle (ed.) *Communication Disorders in Multicultural Populations* (2nd edn; p. 279). Boston: Butterworth-Heinemann.

Dejonckere, P.H., Bradley, P., Clements, P., Cornet, G., Crevier-Buchman, L., Friedrich, G., *et al.* (2001) A basic protocol for functional assessment of voice pathology, especially for investigating the efficacy of (phonosurgical) treatment and evaluating new assessment techniques. *European Archives of Otorhinolaryngology* 258 (2), 77–82.

Hapner, E.R., Portone-Maira, C. and Johns, M.M. (2009) A study of voice therapy drop out. *Journal of Voice* 23 (3), 333–337.

Hirano, M. (1981) *Clinical Examination of the Voice*. New York: Springer-Verlag.

Jacobson, B.H., Johnson, A., Grywalski, C., Silbergleit, A., Jacobson, G., Benninger, M.S., *et al.* (1997) The Voice Handicap Index (VHI): Development and validation. *American Journal of Speech-Language Pathology* 6, 66–70.

Kempster, G.B., Gerratt, B.R., Verdolini Abbott, K., Barkmeier-Kraemer, J. and Hillman, R.E. (2009) Consensus auditory-perceptual evaluation of voice: Development of a standardized clinical protocol. *American Journal of Speech-Language Pathology* 18 (2), 124–132.

Kotby, M.N., El-Sady, S.R., Basiouny, S.E., Abou-Rass, Y.A. and Hegazi, M.A. (1981) The efficacy of the accent method of voice therapy. *Journal of Voice* 5 (4), 316–320.

Kreiman, J., Gerratt, B.R., Kempster, G.B., Erman, A. and Berke, G.S. (1993) Perceptual evaluation of voice quality: Review, tutorial, and a framework for future research. *Journal of Speech and Hearing Research* 36, 21–40.

Ma, E.P.M., Yiu, E.M.L. and Verdolini Abbott, K. (2007) Application of the ICF in voice disorders. *Seminars in Speech and Language* 28 (4), 343–350.

Oates, J. and Russell, A. (1998) Learning voice analysis using an interactive multi-media package: Development and preliminary evaluation. *Journal of Voice* 12, 500–512.

Ramig, L.O., Fox, C. and Sapir, S. (2004) Parkinson's disease: Speech and voice disorders and their treatment with the Lee Silverman Voice Treatment. *Seminars in Speech and Language* 25, 169–180.

Roy, N. and Leeper, H.A. (1993) Effects of the manual laryngeal musculoskeletal tension reduction technique as a treatment for functional voice disorders: Perceptual and acoustic measures. *Journal of Voice* 7, 242–249.

Roy, N., Weinrich, B., Gray, S., Tanner, K., Toledo, S., Dove, H., *et al.* (2002) Voice amplification versus vocal hygiene instruction for teachers with voice disorders: A treatment outcomes study. *Journal of Speech, Language, and Hearing Research* 45, 625–638.

Roy, N., Weinrich, B., Gray, S.D., Tanner, K., Stemple, J.C. and Sapienza, C.M. (2003) Three treatments for teachers with voice disorders: A randomized clinical trial. *Journal of Speech-Language and Hearing Research* 46, 670–688.

Roy, N., Merrill, R.M., Thibeault, S., Parsa, R.A., Gray, S.D. and Smith, E.M. (2004) Prevalence of voice disorders in teachers and the general population. *Journal of Speech, Language, and Hearing Research* 47, 281–293.

Rubin, J.S., Wendler, J., Woisard, V., Dejonckere, P.H., Wellens, W. and Kotby, N. (2007) Phoniatric provision and training: Current European perspectives. *Journal of Laryngology & Otology* 121, 427–430.

Sataloff, R.T., Spiegel, J.R. and Hawkshaw, M.J. (1991) Strobovideolaryngoscopy: Results and clinical value. *Annals of Otology, Rhinology, and Laryngology* 100, 725–727.

Schwartz, S.R., Cohen, S.M., Dailey, S.H., Rosenfeld, R.M., Deutsch, E.S., Gillespie, M.B., *et al.* (2009) Clinical practice guideline: Hoarseness (dysphonia). *Otolaryngology – Head and Neck Surgery* 141, S1–S31.

Stemple, J.C. and Fry, L.T. (2010) *Voice Therapy: Clinical Case Studies* (3rd edn; pp. 2–10). San Diego: Plural Publishing.

Stemple, J., Lee, L., D'Amico, B. and Pickup, B. (1994) Efficacy of vocal function exercises as a method of improving voice production. *Journal of Voice* 8, 271–278.

Thomas, L.B. and Stemple, J.C. (2007) Voice therapy: Does science support the art? *Communicative Disorders Review* 1 (1), 51–79.

van Leer E. and Connor N.P. (2010) Patient perceptions of voice therapy adherence. *Journal of Voice* 24 (4), 458–469.

Verdolini, K. (1998) Resonant voice therapy. In K. Verdolini (ed.) *National Center for Voice and Speech's Guide to Vocology* (pp. 34–35). Iowa City: National Center for Voice and Speech.

WHO (2001) *International Classification of Functioning, Disability, and Health*. Geneva: World Health Organization.

# Part 2

# Contemporary Voice Research:
# A World Perspective

# 10 Contemporary Voice Research in Japan

## Shigeru Hirano

## Introduction

In the past three decades, voice research in Japan has developed rapidly in the field of histology, physiology, imaging and regenerative medicine. Regenerative medicine using tissue engineering to restore laryngeal tissue and its function has received widespread attention.

Minoru Hirano and colleagues (Hirano, 1975; Hirano & Kakita, 1985) led the research into laryngeal anatomy in the 1970s. Their findings contributed in the development of phonosurgery. In addition to research in laryngeal anatomy, aerodynamic and acoustic measurements of phonation have also been studied extensively in the characterization of voice function. Aerodynamic study was first developed by a group of researchers led by Masayuki Sawashima. Maximum phonation time (MPT), mean flow rate (MFR) and subglottic pressure were the major measures that were investigated under aerodynamic studies. Sawashima et al. (1987) developed the momentary airway interruption method as a non-invasive way to measure subglottic pressure without the requirement of the insertion of a needle into the trachea. In this method, the subject was instructed to say /pa/, and intraoral pressure was measured during the phonation as a substitute for subglottic pressure, because intraoral pressure was regarded as the same as subglottic pressure during the articulation of /p/. Kitajima and Fujita (1990) also developed a non-invasive measurement of subglottic pressure using /i:pi:/ phonation.

The investigation of acoustic measurements such as perturbation and noise energy began in the 1960s. The use of pitch perturbation was first reported by Shigenobu Iwata with Hans von Leden (1970), amplitude perturbation was reported by Yasuo Koike (1969), and noise measurements were reported by research groups led by Eiji Yumoto (Yumoto et al., 1982) and Hideki Kasuya (Kasuya et al., 1986). These aerodynamic and acoustic measurements have become the standard voice measurements in clinical voice assessment.

Voice research in recent years has been facilitated by new developments of technology in basic science, imaging apparatus and optical instruments. The advancement of basic science research techniques has also made it possible to develop genomic and proteomic analyses in voice research. For example, gene expression of the extracellular matrix (ECM) in the vocal fold mucosa can now be detected using polymerase chain reaction (PCR) or *in situ* hybridization. These new approaches have shed more light on the understanding of genetics in voice research.

This chapter outlines recent voice research developments in Japan. Three broad areas will be discussed: (1) the anatomy and neurology of the vocal folds; (2) imaging techniques of the vocal folds, and (3) tissue engineering of the larynx.

## Histological Research on Voice

One of the most important histological research findings is the layered structure of the human vocal fold revealed by Minoru Hirano and colleagues (Hirano, 1975; Hirano & Kakita, 1985). They found that the vocal fold consists of an epithelium, three layers of lamina propria and a layer of muscle. The two deeper layers of the lamina propria form the vocal ligament. The unique feature of the different viscoelasticity in each of these layers is essential for the vibratory requirement of the vocal folds (Hirano, 1977). This layered structure is also called the 'cover body' structure, in which the cover is the main vibratory portion consisting of the epithelium and superficial layer of the lamina propria. The development of and aging effects on this layered structure have also been well documented (Hirano et al., 1983).

ECM is the key factor that determines the viscoelasticity of the vocal fold mucosa. Distribution of ECM components has also been reported by Hirano (Hirano, 1977; Hirano & Kakita, 1985) and Sato and colleagues (Sato & Hirano, 1997; Sato et al., 2000). They demonstrated that collagen basically exists in the deep layer of lamina propria, and collagen type III, known as 'reticular fiber', is located in the superficial layer, while elastic fiber is distributed in the intermediate layer (Sato, 1998). Age-related changes of these ECM have also been well documented (Hirano et al., 1989; Sato & Hirano, 1997; Sato et al., 2002). The proportion of collagen fiber increases in aged vocal folds, frequently forming disorganized thick bundles, while elastin and reticular fibers decrease. Alteration of ECM in pathological vocal folds has also been reported (Sato & Hirano, 1998; Sato et al., 1999).

The study of cells in the vocal fold has received much attention since 2000. Hirano and Sato first demonstrated the presence of different types of fibroblasts in the vocal fold mucosa using electron microscopy (Hirano et al., 1999, 2000; Sato et al., 2001). They found that the fibroblast in the macula flava is different from that in Reinke's space in terms of shape, density and superstructure. The type of fibroblasts in the macula flava are called 'stellate cells' because they have stellate shapes, while fibroblasts in Reinke's space take the shape of spindles. Stellate cells have rich intracellular organelles including Golgi apparatus, rough endoplasmic reticulum (rER) and mitochondria. The development of these organelles means high vitality and ability to produce the proteins of ECM, which has led to the hypothesis that stellate cells may contribute to the metabolism and maintenance of the vocal fold mucosa. On the other hand, it was confirmed that stellate cells can produce hyaluronic acid (HA), which is regarded as the most important ECM for vibratory property (Sato et al., 2006). Stellate cells are more developed in humans as compared to other animals (Sato et al., 2000). Another remarkable aspect of stellate cells is the storage of vitamin A inside the cytoplasm. Vitamin A plays an important role in organogenesis, and it also contributes to maintaining collagen. Recently Tateya et al. (2008) demonstrated that vitamin A may work in controlling collagen type I in the vocal fold mucosa, using vitamin A-deficient rats. Sato et al. (2008) also indicated that, in irradiated vocal folds, stellate cells are degenerated causing a decrease in activity to maintain the mucosa, which may lead to fibrotic changes after radiation. A comprehensive summary of the role of the macula flava was published in 2010 by Sato et al. (2010a, 2010b).

# Neurolaryngology

Neurolaryngology is another area that has been widely researched in Japan for more than 30 years. One of the most significant studies was conducted by Minoru Hirano and Yoshikazu Yoshida to investigate the central nervous control of the larynx using a retrograde nerve tracer in the 1980s. They used horseradish peroxidase (HRP) as a nerve tracer and found that the nerve in the intrinsic laryngeal muscle fibers projected up to the nucleus ambiguous in the medulla in cats and monkeys (Yoshida et al., 1982, 1984, 1985). Around the same time, Yasuo Hisa and colleagues studied the recurrent laryngeal nerve of rats using WGA-HRP (Hisa et al., 1985). Later they used another new tracer, cholera toxin subunit B-conjugated gold (CTBG) to examine the roles of several neurotransmitters in canine laryngeal sensory innervations (Hisa et al., 1994). Their studies include the investigations of laryngeal innervations in the motor, sensory and autonomic nervous system using immunohistochemistry and the labeling technique mentioned above. Their findings on neurotransmitters and neuromodulators involved in laryngeal innervation were summarized and reported in 1999 (Hisa et al., 1999).

Research into neurolaryngology in the 21st century has extended into the study of the role of nitric oxide, capsaicin and growth factor. Hisa and colleagues examined the role of nitric oxide after injury of the recurrent laryngeal nerve by revealing the expression of nitric oxide synthase in the nucleus ambiguus using immunohistochemistry. The possible role of nitric oxide during nerve injury was demonstrated (Bamba *et al.*, 2000). They also investigated the expression of fibroblast growth factor-1 (FGF1) in the motor nucleus of the vagus nerve in rats (Okano *et al.*, 2006), and found that FGF1 is localized at the motor neurons, postganglionic parasympathetic neurons and sensory neurons, with relatively low expression in the preganglionic parasympathetic cholinergic neurons. Their results supported the notion that cholingergic neurons in the dorsal motor nucleus of the vagus (DMNV) are particularly vulnerable to laryngeal nerve damage, possibly because of the lack of FGF1.

A recent research area concerns circadian gene expression in the larynx (Nishio *et al.*, 2008). The circadian expression of mPer1, mPer2, C/EBPbeta, HNF3beta, and MUC5b using adult wild-type C57/B16 mice and mCry1(-/-) mCry2(-/-) mutant mice by immunohistochemistry and/or Northern blotting were examined. They found that the expression of mPer2 mRNA showed a strong day–night expression difference in mCry1(-/-) mCry2(-/-) mutant mice. They also found that mPER1 and mPER2 proteins both showed very similar expression profiles in the epithelium and submucosal glands, with a peak in the evening and a trough in the early morning. MUC5b protein also showed circadian oscillation in the laryngeal submucosal gland. Nishio *et al.* (2008) suggested that these rhythmic expressions may cause the time-specific symptoms among laryngeal diseases.

Researchers from Asahikawa Medical School have conducted a series of studies on the voice-related region of the brain. Nonaka *et al.* (1999) found that electrical stimulation to the periaqueductal gray (PAG) evoked vocalization in decerebrated cats. Akihiro Katada further examined the positive effects of electrical stimulation to PAG on the improvement of voice in cats with recurrent laryngeal damage (Katada *et al.*, 2004). Hisa and colleagues recently conducted a study on the systematic electrical and chemical stimulation of the brainstem in guinea pigs to identify the similarities in the call sites between murines and other mammals (Sugiyama *et al.*, 2010). They found that the brainstem call areas and vocal motor patterns induced from these samples were approximately consistent with those in other mammals.

# Research on Vocal Fold Vibration Using High-speed Digital Imaging

High-speed imaging of the vocal fold vibration has been of great interest for the visualization of real-time vibratory motion ever since Minoru Hirano reported on the prototype of high-speed equipment in 1974 (Hirano *et al.*, 1974). The prototype was gigantic and allowed black-and-white images only. Later at Tokyo University, a new method of digital imaging of vocal fold vibration using a solid-state image sensor attached to a conventional camera system was developed (Hirose, 1988). The maximum frame rate for analysis was 4000 fps. The system is useful for clinical examination of pathological vocal fold vibration.

More recently, the Tokyo University group reported two other image analysis systems using videokymographic and laryngotopographic methods. Laryngotopographic analysis of unilateral vocal fold paralysis (UVFP) revealed two distinct frequencies of vibration for the paralyzed vocal fold and the contralateral intact vocal folds (Kimura et al., 2010a, 2010b). There is a stereotactic high-speed digital imaging technique study in progress to investigate three-dimensional visualization of vocal fold vibration.

Sekimoto et al. (2009) developed a special purpose adaptor, making it possible to use a commercially available high-speed camera to observe vocal fold vibration during phonation. Although the frame rate is at 1200 cycles per second only, the cost of the system is relatively low and this makes the availability of high-speed in clinical practice more affordable (Sekimoto et al., 2009).

# Laryngeal Imaging

Recent imaging systems such as three-dimensional computed tomography (3D-CT) and magnetic resonance imaging (MRI) have also been applied to laryngeal imaging. Eiji Yumoto and colleagues (Yumoto et al., 1997) first succeeded in obtaining 3D-CT images of the larynx during phonation using a helical CT and multiplanner reconstruction (MPR) method. This technique provided 3D-CT endoscopic images of the internal lumen of the larynx. They showed data of normal subjects and patients with paralysis and atrophy. The images can be obtained in 5 seconds during phonation by a high-speed data acquisition system (Yumoto et al., 2003). Their findings showed that 84% of paralyzed vocal folds were thinner than normal vocal folds and 57% of them positioned their larynges higher than the normal vocal folds. Bowing, level difference, overadduction and paradoxical movement were clearly detected by the CT analysis (Yumoto, 2004).

Recently, Hiramatsu and colleagues developed a 3D-CT laryngeal model, with helical CT and MIMICS software (Materialize Japan Co, Yokohama) analyzing programs, which enables motion analysis of the vocal folds and arytenoids cartilage (Hiramatsu et al., 2006, 2009). They examined the characteristics of 3D arytenoids movement in 61 subjects with UVFP. The cricoid and arytenoid cartilages were examined by 3D-CT and the movements of the paralyzed vocal folds were compared during quiet inspiration and phonation. The results found that 90.7% of cases demonstrated passive gliding movement of the paralyzed arytenoids. This correlated with the worsening of MFR. They concluded that the degree of the displacement of the arytenoids is one indicator that can be used to evaluate the severity of UVFP.

A three-dimensional cine-MRI technique based on a synchronized sampling method was developed by ATR (Advanced Telecommunications Research Institute International) Human Information Science Laboratories (Takemoto et al., 2006). The system measured the temporal changes in the vocal tract area during the production of a short utterance (/aiueo/) in Japanese. A time series of head-neck volumes was obtained after 64 repetitions of the utterances, from which area functions were extracted frame by frame. A region-based analysis showed that the volumes of the anterior and posterior portions of oral cavities tend to change reciprocally and that the areas near the larynx and posterior edge of the hard palate were almost constant throughout the utterances.

## Regenerative Medicine of the Larynx

Regenerative medicine with tissue engineering was the breakthrough in the late 20th century in a number of medical fields. This innovative technology has also been applied to laryngeal regeneration. Regenerative medicine targets histologically altered laryngeal tissues, particularly the vocal folds, to restore the vibratory and respiratory properties. This technology also aims to regenerate the hemilarynx or total larynx, and in some cases the whole cartilage, muscle and mucosa tissues for the restoration of laryngeal function after laryngectomy. Tissue engineering has three important elements: cells, scaffolding and growth factors. Appropriate use and/or a combination of these elements are important factors in regeneration.

The research group at Kyoto University has obtained significant achievements in their research on laryngeal regeneration. Cell therapy has been used for tissue regeneration and Shigeru Hirano and colleagues first reported the use of vocal fold fibroblasts to restore scarred canine vocal folds (Hirano et al., 2004b). The results were, however, unsuccessful as the vocal folds treated by the injection of autologous fibroblasts were still severely scarred. They reported that it was difficult to correctly control the mature fibroblasts in vivo. They have switched to the use of immature cells such as stem cells. More recently, Shin-ichi Kanemaru and colleagues developed cell culture systems of bone marrow-derived stem cell (MSC) (Kanemaru et al., 2003a, 2005), and treated injured canine vocal folds by injection of MSC. The results were encouraging, which demonstrated better tissue recovery of the injured vocal folds. It was contended that the injected MSCs had multipotency as they developed into several tissue types including the epithelium, muscle and mesenchymal tissues. Stem cell therapy has a great potential for laryngeal regeneration. However, clinical application of stem cell therapy is still in its infancy because of a number of ethical and legal issues.

Growth factor therapy is another effective strategy in tissue engineering, in which growth factors are applied to local sites or systemically to regenerate tissues. Exogenous growth factor is thought to be a trigger to stimulate cells and modulate their functions by changing the phenotype. It triggers healing processes and induces tissue regeneration. Growth factors can be applied in several ways, such as a single injection, repeated injections or by using a drug delivery system. Therefore, a simple application of solution of growth factor still has regenerative effects but, for refractory cases, repeated applications or through drug delivery systems are used to strengthen the effects. Shigeru Hirano and colleagues have extensively researched hepatocyte growth factor (HGF) and basic fibroblast growth factor (bFGF) for the regeneration of the vocal folds. They examined the effects of HGF and vocal fold fibroblasts *in vitro*, and revealed that HGF stimulated the production of HA and suppressed collagen synthesis from the fibroblasts (Hirano *et al.*, 2003a, 2003b, 2003c). These biological effects were regarded as appropriate for restoring vocal fold functions. Kishimoto *et al.* (2009) further confirmed that exogenous HGF stimulated the production of endogenous HGF in vocal fold cells, suggesting an autocrine loop of HGF. Subsequent animal studies using rabbits and dogs showed remarkable regenerative effects of HGF for the prevention and treatment of scarred vocal folds (Hirano *et al.*, 2004b, 2004c). The group developed a novel drug delivery system for HGF using gelatin hydrogel, in which HGF was control-released *in vivo* over 2 weeks. This drug delivery system has proved to be useful for treating not only acute scar but also chronic scar of the vocal folds (Kishimoto *et al.*, 2010; Ohno *et al.*, 2007). Recently, HGF has also been found to be effective for aged vocal fold atrophy (T. Ohno *et al.*, 2009a).

The Kyoto team has also examined bFGF as a therapeutic potential for aged vocal fold atrophy by *in vitro* and *in vivo* set ups. Hirano and colleagues reported that bFGF stimulated HA production from aged rat vocal fold fibroblasts, and then confirmed its regenerative effects by injecting bFGF into aged rat vocal folds (Hirano *et al.*, 2004a, 2005). T. Ohno *et al.* (2009b) further examined the effects at the genetic level using PCR. They found that bFGF upregulated hyaluronic acid synthase (HAS) 2, 3, and matrix metalloproteinase-2 (MMP-2) in aged rat vocal folds. Hirano and colleagues set up a clinical trial of treatment of aged vocal fold atrophy with localized injection of bFGF product, and the first case was reported in 2008 with positive results indicating improved vibratory property and better voice quality after administration of bFGF (Hirano *et al.*, 2008). Recently his colleague also attempted to treat vocal fold scars by using bFGF and showed a good restoration of canine scarred vocal folds (Suehiro *et al.*, 2010). In conclusion, therapeutic effects of both HGF and bFGF have been confirmed for either scarred or atrophied vocal folds.

The Kyoto team has also conducted research on laryngeal regeneration using 'scaffolding'. The concept of scaffolding is to provide an appropriate temporary space for regeneration. An ideal regenerative scaffold is biocompatible, biodegradable and attracts cells around the place to influx into the scaffold. For this purpose several materials have been developed, such as HA hydrogel, acellular ECM, collagen or gelatin sponge. In Japan, Hirano and colleagues have examined the feasibility of bovine-derived atelocollagen sponge, usable to humans in Japan, as a scaffold that provides a place of regeneration of tissues, using *in vitro* set ups (S. Ohno *et al.*, 2009). MSCs from rats were cultured on the scaffold, and the cells were found to survive and proliferate, producing fibronectin. The research group implanted the material into scarred vocal folds or sulcus vocalis in six individuals (Kishimoto *et al.*, 2009). Their results showed gradual improvement of the acoustic parameters of voice over six months, although individual variation was noted. More effective strategies to induce regeneration with the scaffold are still being developed.

Yamashita *et al.* (2010) attempted to regenerate tissues after hemi-laryngectomy using implantation of polypropylene collagen mesh. They implanted the material to the defect after hemilaryngectomy of canine, and showed positive regenerative effects with re-epithelialization on the inner lumen. However, the need to explore more appropriate materials is warranted because foreign body reaction or infection has been observed in some individuals. Scaffolding is most feasible for clinical application, but its regenerative effects are limited. It may well be necessary to combine its use with growth factors and/or cells to induce a better regeneration of tissues.

Koichi Omori and colleagues at the Fukushima Medical School have intensively conducted research on developing artificial trachea using polypropylene and collagen mesh for tracheal regeneration (Nomoto *et al.*, 2006; Omori *et al.*, 2005). After confirming biocompatibility and the regenerative effects of the implant material to treat tracheal defects of canine, they applied the material to human cases who underwent tracheal resection because of thyroid cancer. The first successful case was reported in 2005 (Omori *et al.*, 2005). In the meantime, they also applied the same material to regenerate the cricoid cartilage in canine, which also showed successful reconstruction of the framework with sufficient re-epithelialization (Omori *et al.*, 2004).

Regeneration of recurrent laryngeal nerve was attempted by Kanemaru and colleagues using a polyglycolic acid (PGA) tube (Kanemaru *et al.*, 2003b). They interposed the tube between both ends of the canine recurrent laryngeal nerve after resection of the nerve of 2 cm in length. The nerve fibers were well regenerated through the tube, and recovery of the movement of the treated vocal folds was clearly demonstrated.

In summary, Japanese researchers have worked on several aspects including histology, neurolaryngology and development of acoustic and aerodynamic measurements, as well as imaging systems. Lately, research on regenerative medicine for the larynx have received more and more attention in treating altered histology of the vocal folds such as atrophy, scarring and sulcus, as well as in reconstructing defects after partial laryngectomy.

# References

Bamba, H., Uno, T., Koike, S., Shogaki, K. and Hisa, Y. (2000) Induction of nitric oxide synthase activity in nucleus ambiguus motoneurons after injury to the rat recurrent laryngeal nerve. *Acta Oto-laryngologica* 120 (2), 327–329.

Hiramatsu, H., Tokashiki, R., Yamaguchi, H., Suzuki, M. and Ono, H. (2006) Three-dimensional laryngeal model for planning of laryngeal framework surgery. *Acta Oto-laryngologica* 126 (5), 515–520.

Hiramatsu, H., Tokashiki, R., Nakamura, M., Motohashi, R., Yoshida, T. and Suzuki, M. (2009) Characterization of arytenoid vertical displacement in unilateral vocal fold paralysis by three-dimensional computed tomography. *European Archives of Oto-Rhino-Laryngology* 266 (1), 97–104.

Hirano, M. (1975) Phonosurgery: Basic and clinical investigations. *Otologia (Fukuoka)* 21, 239–440.

Hirano, M. (1977) Structure and vibratory behavior of the vocal folds. In M. Sawashima and F. Cooper (eds) *Dynamic Aspects of Speech Production* (pp. 13–30). Tokyo: University of Tokyo.

Hirano, M. and Kakita, Y. (1985) Cover-body theory of vocal fold vibration. In R.G. Daniloff (ed.) *Speech Science* (pp. 1–46). San Diego: College-Hill Press.

Hirano, M., Yoshida, Y., Matsushita, H. and Nakashima, T. (1974) An apparatus for ultra-high-speed cinematography of the vocal folds. *Annals of Otology, Rhinology, and Laryngology* 83 (1), 12–18.

Hirano, M., Kurita, S. and Nakashima, T. (1983) Growth, development and aging of human vocal folds. In D.M. Bless and J.H. Abbs (eds) *Vocal Fold Physiology* (pp. 22–43). San Diego: College-Hill Press.

Hirano, M., Kurita, S. and Sakaguchi, S. (1989) Ageing of the vibratory tissue of human vocal folds. *Acta Oto-laryngologica* 107 (5–6), 428–433.

Hirano, M., Sato, K. and Nakashima, T. (1999) Fibroblasts in human vocal fold mucosa. *Acta Oto-laryngologica* 119 (2), 271–276.

Hirano, M., Sato, K. and Nakashima, T. (2000) Fibroblasts in geriatric vocal fold mucosa. *Acta Oto-laryngologica* 120 (2), 336–340.

Hirano, S., Bless, D.M., Heisey, D. and Ford, C.N. (2003a) Effect of growth factors on hyaluronan production by canine vocal fold fibroblasts. *Annals of Otology, Rhinology, and Laryngology* 112 (7), 617–624.

Hirano, S., Bless, D.M., Heisey, D. and Ford, C.N. (2003b) Roles of hepatocyte growth factor and transforming growth factor β1 in production of extracellular matrix by canine vocal fold fibroblasts. *Laryngoscope* 113 (1), 144–148.

Hirano, S., Bless, D.M., Massey, R.J., Hartig, G.K. and Ford, C.N. (2003c) Morphological and functional changes of human vocal fold fibroblasts with hepatocyte growth factor. *Annals of Otology, Rhinology, and Laryngology* 112 (12), 1026–1033.

Hirano, S., Bless, D.M., del Río, A.M., Connor, N.P. and Ford, C.N. (2004a) Therapeutic potential of growth factors for aging voice. *Laryngoscope* 114 (12), 2161–2167.

Hirano, S., Bless, D.M., Nagai, H., Rousseau, B., Welham, N.V., Montequin, D.W., *et al.* (2004b) Growth factor therapy for vocal fold scarring in a canine model. *Annals of Otology, Rhinology, and Laryngology* 113 (10), 777–785.

Hirano, S., Bless, D.M., Rousseau, B., Welham, N., Montequin, D., Chan, R.W., *et al.* (2004c) Prevention of vocal fold scarring by topical injection of hepatocyte growth factor in a rabbit model. *Laryngoscope* 114 (3), 548–556.

Hirano, S., Nagai, H., Tateya, I., Tateya, T., Ford, C.N. and Bless, D.M. (2005) Regeneration of aged vocal folds with basic fibroblast growth factor in a rat model: A preliminary report. *Annals of Otology, Rhinology, and Laryngology* 114 (4), 304–308.

Hirano, S., Kishimoto, Y., Suehiro, A., Kanemaru, S.-i. and Ito, J. (2008) Regeneration of aged vocal fold: First human case treated with fibroblast growth factor. *Laryngoscope* 118 (12), 2254–2259.

Hirose, H. (1988) High-speed digital imaging of vocal fold vibration. *Acta Oto-laryngologica* 105 (s458), 151–153.

Hisa, Y., Lyon, M.J. and Malmgren, L.T. (1985) Central projection of the sensory component of the rat recurrent laryngeal nerve. *Neuroscience Letters* 55 (2), 185–190.

Hisa, Y., Tadaki, N., Uno, T., Okamura, H., Taguchi, J. and Ibata, Y. (1994) Neuropeptide participation in canine laryngeal sensory innervation. Immunohistochemistry and retrograde labeling. *Annals of Otology, Rhinology, and Laryngology* 103 (10), 767–770.

Hisa, Y., Koike, S., Tadaki, N., Bamba, H., Shogaki, K. and Uno, T. (1999) Neurotransmitters and neuromodulators involved in laryngeal innervation. *Annals of Otology, Rhinology, and Laryngology* Suppl. 178, 3–14.

Iwata, S. and von Leden, H. (1970) Pitch perturbations in normal and pathologic voices. *Folia Phoniatrica et Logopaedica* 22 (6), 413–424.

Kanemaru, S., Nakamura, T., Omori, K., Kojima, H., Magrufov, A., Hiratsuka, Y., *et al.* (2003a) Regeneration of the vocal fold using autologous mesenchymal stem cells. *Annals of Otology, Rhinology, and Laryngology* 112 (11), 915–920.

Kanemaru, S., Nakamura, T., Omori, K., Kojima, H., Magrufov, A., Hiratsuka, Y., *et al.* (2003b) Recurrent laryngeal nerve regeneration by tissue engineering. *Annals of Otology, Rhinology, and Laryngology* 112 (6), 492–498.

Kanemaru, S., Nakamura, T., Yamashita, M., Magrufov, A., Kita, T., Tamaki, H., *et al.* (2005) Destiny of autologous bone marrow-derived stromal cells implanted in the vocal fold. *Annals of Otology, Rhinology, and Laryngology* 114 (12), 907–912.

Kasuya, H., Ogawa, S., Mashima, K. and Ebihara, S. (1986) Normalized noise energy as an acoustic measure to evaluate pathologic voice. *Journal of the Acoustical Society of America* 80 (5), 1329–1334.

Katada, A., Nonaka, S., Adachi, M., Kunibe, I., Arakawa, T., Imada, M., *et al.* (2004) Functional electrical stimulation of laryngeal adductor muscle restores mobility of vocal fold and improves voice sounds in cats with unilateral laryngeal paralysis. *Neuroscience Research* 50 (2), 153–159.

Kimura, M., Imagawa, H., Nito, T., Sakakibara, K., Chan, R.W. and Tayama, N. (2010a) Arytenoid adduction for correcting vocal fold asymmetry: High-speed imaging. *Annals of Otology, Rhinology, and Laryngology* 119 (7), 439–446.

Kimura, M., Nito, T., Imagawa, H., Sakakibara, K., Chan, R.W. and Tayama, N. (2010b) Collagen injection for correcting vocal fold asymmetry: High-speed imaging. *Annals of Otology, Rhinology, and Laryngology* 119 (6), 359–368.

Kishimoto, Y., Hirano, S., Suehiro, A., Tateya, I., Kanemaru, S., Nakamura, T., *et al.* (2009) Effect of exogenous hepatocyte growth factor on vocal fold fibroblasts. *Annals of Otology, Rhinology, and Laryngology* 118 (8), 606–611.

Kishimoto, Y., Hirano, S., Kitani, Y., Suehiro, A., Umeda, H., Tateya, I., *et al.* (2010) Chronic vocal fold scar restoration with hepatocyte growth factor hydrogel. *Laryngoscope* 120 (1), 108–113.

Kitajima, K. and Fujita, F. (1990) Estimation of subglottal pressure with intraoral pressure. *Acta Oto-laryngologica* 109 (5–6), 473–478.

Koike, Y. (1969) Vowel amplitude modulations in patients with laryngeal diseases. *Journal of the Acoustical Society of America* 45 (4), 839–844.

Nishio, T., Bando, H., Bamba, H., Hisa, Y. and Okamura, H. (2008) Circadian gene expression in the murine larynx. *Auris Nasus Larynx* 35 (4), 539–544.

Nomoto, Y., Suzuki, T., Tada, Y., Kobayashi, K., Miyake, M., Hazama, A., *et al.* (2006) Tissue engineering for regeneration of the tracheal epithelium. *Annals of Otology, Rhinology, and Laryngology* 115 (7), 501–506.

Nonaka, S., Katada, A., Sakamoto, T. and Unno, T. (1999) Brain stem neural mechanisms for vocalization in decerebrate cats. *Annals of Otology, Rhinology, and Laryngology* Suppl. 178, 15–24.

Ohno, S., Hirano, S., Tateya, I., Kanemaru, S., Umeda, H., Suehiro, A., *et al.* (2009) Atelocollagen sponge as a stem cell implantation scaffold for the treatment of scarred vocal folds. *Annals of Otology, Rhinology, and Laryngology* 118 (11), 805–810.

Ohno, T., Hirano, S., Kanemaru, S., Yamashita, M., Umeda, H., Suehiro, A., *et al.* (2007) Drug delivery system of hepatocyte growth factor for the treatment of vocal fold scarring in a canine model. *Annals of Otology, Rhinology, and Laryngology* 116 (10), 762–769.

Ohno, T., Yoo, M.J., Swanson, E.R., Hirano, S., Ossoff, R.H. and Rousseau, B. (2009a) Regeneration of aged rat vocal folds using hepatocyte growth factor therapy. *Laryngoscope* 119 (7), 1424–1430.

Ohno, T., Yoo, M.J., Swanson, E.R., Hirano, S., Ossoff, R.H. and Rousseau, B. (2009b) Regenerative effects of basic fibroblast growth factor on extracellular matrix production in aged rat vocal folds. *Annals of Otology, Rhinology, and Laryngology* 118 (8), 559–564.

Okano, H., Toyoda, K., Bamba, H., Hisa, Y., Oomura, Y., Imamura, T., *et al.* (2006) Localization of fibroblast growth factor-1 in cholinergic neurons innervating the rat larynx. *Journal of Histochemistry & Cytochemistry* 54 (9), 1061–1071.

Omori, K., Nakamura, T., Kanemaru, S., Kojima, H., Magrufov, A., Hiratsuka, Y., *et al.* (2004) Cricoid regeneration using in situ tissue engineering in canine larynx for the treatment of subglottic stenosis. *Annals of Otology, Rhinology, and Laryngology* 113 (8), 623–627.

Omori, K., Nakamura, T., Kanemaru, S., Asato, R., Yamashita, M., Tanaka, S., *et al.* (2005) Regenerative medicine of the trachea: The first human case. *Annals of Otology, Rhinology, and Laryngology* 114 (6), 429–433.

Sato, K. (1998) Reticular fibers in the vocal fold mucosa. *Annals of Otology, Rhinology, and Laryngology* 107 (12), 1023–1028.

Sato, K. and Hirano, M. (1997) Age-related changes of elastic fibers in the superficial layer of the lamina propria of vocal folds. *Annals of Otology, Rhinology, and Laryngology* 106 (1), 44–48.

Sato, K. and Hirano, M. (1998) Electron microscopic investigation of sulcus vocalis. *Annals of Otology, Rhinology, and Laryngology* 107 (1), 56–60.

Sato, K., Hirano, M. and Nakashima, T. (1999) Electron microscopic and immunohistochemical investigation of Reinke's edema. *Annals of Otology, Rhinology, and Laryngology* 108 (11, Part 1), 1068–1072.

Sato, K., Hirano, M. and Nakashima, T. (2000) Comparative histology of the maculae flavae of the vocal folds. *Annals of Otology, Rhinology, and Laryngology* 109 (2), 136–140.

Sato, K., Hirano, M. and Nakashima, T. (2001) Stellate cells in the human vocal fold. *Annals of Otology, Rhinology, and Laryngology* 110 (4), 319–325.

Sato, K., Hirano, M. and Nakashima, T. (2002) Age-related changes of collagenous fibers in the human vocal fold mucosa. *Annals of Otology, Rhinology, and Laryngology* 111 (1), 15–20.

Sato, K., Sakamoto, K. and Nakashima, T. (2006) Expression and distribution of CD44 and hyaluronic acid in human vocal fold mucosa. *Annals of Otology, Rhinology, and Laryngology* 115 (10), 741–748.

Sato, K., Shirouzu, H. and Nakashima, T. (2008) Irradiated macula flava in the human vocal fold mucosa. *American Journal of Otolaryngology* 29 (5), 312–318.

Sato, K., Umeno, H. and Nakashima, T. (2010a) Functional histology of the macula flava in the human vocal fold – part 1: Its role in the adult vocal fold. *Folia Phoniatrica et Logopaedica* 62 (4), 178–184.

Sato, K., Umeno, H. and Nakashima, T. (2010b) Functional histology of the macula flava in the human vocal fold – part 2: Its role in the growth and development of the vocal fold. *Folia Phoniatrica et Logopaedica* 62 (6), 263–270.

Sawashima, M., Honda, K. and Aoki, S. (1987) Use of the airway interruption method for evaluating aerodynamic conditions in phonation. *Japan Journal of Logopedics and Phoniatrics* 28, 257–264.

Sekimoto, S., Tsunoda, K., Kaga, K., Makiyama, K., Tsunoda, A., Kondo, K., *et al.* (2009) Commercially available high-speed system for recording and monitoring vocal fold vibrations. *Acta Oto-laryngologica* 129 (12), 1524–1526.

Suehiro, A., Hirano, S., Kishimoto, Y., Rousseau, B., Nakamura, T. and Ito, J. (2010) Treatment of acute vocal fold scar with local injection of basic fibroblast growth factor: A canine study. *Acta Oto-laryngologica* 130 (7), 844–850.

Sugiyama, Y., Shiba, K., Nakazawa, K., Suzuki, T. and Hisa, Y. (2010) Brainstem vocalization area in guinea pigs. *Neuroscience Research* 66 (4), 359–365.

Takemoto, H., Honda, K., Masaki, S., Shimada, Y. and Fujimoto, I. (2006) Measurement of temporal changes in vocal tract area function from 3D cine-MRI data. *Journal of the Acoustical Society of America* 119 (2), 1037–1049.

Tateya, T., Tateya, I., Surles, R.L., Tanumihardjo, S. and Bless, D.M. (2008) Roles of vitamin A and macula flava in maintaining vocal folds. *Annals of Otology, Rhinology, and Laryngology* 117 (1), 65–73.

Yamashita, M., Kanemaru, S., Hirano, S., Umeda, H., Kitani, Y., Omori, K., *et al.* (2010) Glottal reconstruction with a tissue engineering technique using polypropylene mesh: A canine experiment. *Annals of Otology, Rhinology, and Laryngology* 119 (2), 110–117.

Yoshida, Y., Miyazaki, T., Hirano, M., Shin, T. and Kanaseki, T. (1982) Arrangement of motoneurons innervating the intrinsic laryngeal muscles of cats as demonstrated by horseradish peroxidase. *Acta Oto-laryngologica* 94 (1–6), 329–334.

Yoshida, Y., Mitsumasu, T., Miyazaki, T., Hirano, M. and Kanaseki, T. (1984) Distribution of motoneurons in the brain stem of monkeys, innervating the larynx. *Brain Research Bulletin* 13 (3), 413–419.

Yoshida, Y., Mitsumasu, T., Hirano, M. and Kanaseki, T. (1985) Somatotopic representation of the laryngeal motoneurons in the medulla of monkeys. *Acta Oto-laryngologica* 100 (3–4), 299–303.

Yumoto, E. (2004) Aerodynamics, voice quality, and laryngeal image analysis of normal and pathologic voices. *Current Opinion in Otolaryngology & Head & Neck Surgery* 12 (3), 166–173.

Yumoto, E., Gould, W.J. and Baer, T. (1982) Harmonics-to-noise ratio as an index of the degree of hoarseness. *Journal of the Acoustical Society of America* 71 (6), 1544–1550.

Yumoto, E., Sanuki, T., Hyodo, M., Yasuhara, Y. and Ochi, T. (1997) Three-dimensional endoscopic mode for observation of laryngeal structures by helical computed tomography. *Laryngoscope* 107 (11), 1530–1537.

Yumoto, E., Nakano, K. and Oyamada, Y. (2003) Relationship between 3D behavior of the unilaterally paralyzed larynx and aerodynamic vocal function *Acta Oto-laryngologica* 123 (2), 274–278.

# 11 A USA Perspective: Vocal Fold Injuries and Their Management

## Nicole Yee-Key Li and Katherine Verdolini Abbott

Clinical voice research has been a mainstream research paradigm in the United States. Such an approach plays an important role in evaluating the risk-benefit of a voice treatment for a particular voice-affected population at large. At the same time, in the last two decades, vocal fold biology and tissue engineering have become a critical component of voice research, to advance our understanding of the underlying mechanisms of vocal fold injury and wound healing, as well as in the development of effective and targeted treatment for a range of vocal fold diseases. In this chapter, we will first describe the general principle of wound healing, followed by the current understanding of vocal fold healing mechanisms in two forms of mechanical trauma, namely phonotrauma and surgical trauma, along with their contemporary management approaches. The specific voice studies discussed herein are primarily from research laboratories in the United States unless otherwise stated.

## Overview of Wound Healing

Wound healing is a complex process involving multiple time-dependent interactions among cells, soluble mediators and extracellular matrix (ECM). The normal healing process can be characterized by the following overlapping phases: (1) inflammation; (2) matrix cell migration and proliferation; (3) tissue repair (epithelization, fibroplasia and angiogenesis) and (4) wound remodeling (Mast, 1992; Stadelmann et al., 1998). An alteration of this orderly sequence of events can lead to a chronic wound, such as fibrosis or chronic ulcers. Figure 11.1 describes the cells and the ECM components involved in wound healing.

Inflammation is the earliest and necessary response in wound healing (Hardy, 1989). The inflammatory response results in a vascular response, cellular and fluid exudates, and phagocytic activation in the wound site.

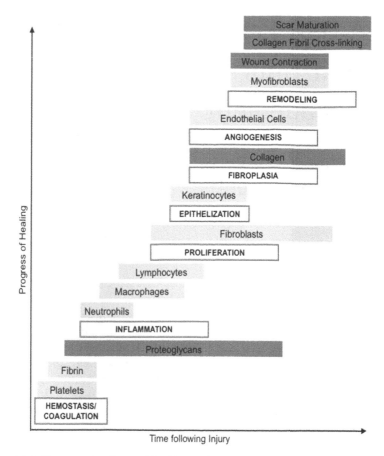

**Figure 11.1** The process of wound healing and the relating cell types and extracellular matrix components

The effects of inflammation can both be beneficial and detrimental. The exudates help to dilute the toxins and the fibrin clots provide a mechanical barrier to the spread of bacteria. Also, the increase in blood flow helps to remove the waste products and increases local oxygen and nutrient supply for cell metabolism, especially for the later proliferative phase. At the same time, the exudates results in edema. The free radicals and lysosomal enzymes produced during phagocytosis may also cause damage to the cell membrane.

During the migratory and proliferative phrases, epithelial cells, fibroblasts and endothelial cells are recruited into the wound site to undergo active mitosis (Hunt *et al.*, 2000). The proliferation of these cells is stimulated by various cytokines and growth factors in the fibrin clot that is formed during the earlier hemostasis/coagulation phase. Once the cells migrate to the wound area, the process of tissue repair starts. Epithelial cells are the primary cells in the process of *epithelization* to re-establish the morphology of the epithelium. Epithelization aims to resume the barrier functions of the epithelium against infection and fluid losses. On the other hand, fibroblasts are the predominant cells in the process of *fibroplasia* to synthesize ECM components in order to repair the connective tissue of the wound. Furthermore, endothelial cells play a role in the process of *angiogenesis* to form new capillaries (Calvin, 1998; Witte & Barbul, 1997). Epithelization is resurfacing a wound with new epithelium (Santoro & Gaudino, 2005), fibroplasia is the formation of fibrous tissue to repair the wound, and angiogenesis is the reconstitution of the blood supply to the wound (Hunt *et al.*, 2000). Epithelization, fibroplasia and angiogenesis are the three processes that start to define the ultimate structure of the scar. The dynamics of these processes are also affected by the available metabolic substrates, tissue oxygen concentration and growth factors during healing (Hunt *et al.*, 2000).

Wound remodeling is the process of reorganization of the neo-matrix patterns in the wound site, which leads to the transition of granulation tissue to a mature scar. Remodeling is the last phase of wound healing, which consists of the processes of wound contraction and ECM reorganization. The remodeling process is initiated while the formation of granulation tissue is progressing. Initially the wound matrix is composed of numerous cells and capillaries and minimal collagen resulting from angiogenesis. Subsequently, during fibroplasia, fibroblasts synthesize and deposit collagen at the wound site. Once a collagen-rich matrix is formed at the wound site, active cell migration stops, inflammatory cells undergo apoptosis and devascularisation starts. Therefore, with maturity, the scar tissue becomes less cellular and vascular but more fibrotic (Calvin, 1998).

# Vocal Fold Injury and Healing

The vocal folds, which are housed in the larynx, have the distinctive geometry, histology and viscoelasticity required for efficient oscillation during phonation (Gray, 2000; Gray *et al.*, 1993, 1994, 2000; Hirano, 1977, 1981; Hirano & Kakita, 1985; Hirano & Sato, 1993; Hirano *et al.*, 1981). The integrity of the vocal fold micro-architecture is critical for proper vocal fold vibration to generate proper voice quality. Such integrity can be disturbed by various sources, such as mechanical trauma as well as chemical or thermal irritation. Depending on the type and magnitude of the disturbance, a range of inflammatory and healing tissue responses will be induced within the vocal fold mucosa, resulting in a regenerative or scarring outcome.

## Phonotraumatic lesions

Phonotrauma is induced by biomechanical stress during phonation. The human vocal folds vibrate naturally at frequencies of 100–1000 Hz and amplitudes of about 1 mm (Titze, 1989). A study reports that teachers turn their voices on and off about 1800 times an hour at work and accumulate up to about 20,000 times a day (Titze et al., 2007). Various mechanical stresses, namely, tensile, contractile, aerodynamic, inertia, impact and shear stresses, act on the mucosa and/or muscles of the vocal folds during phonation (Gunter, 2003, 2004). Pertinent data suggest that phonatory stresses may (1) alter the tissue's physical structure by disrupting intracellular adhesion and cellular structure (Gray & Titze, 1988; Gray et al., 1987), and/or (2) elicit the tissue's biological responses by altering the gene expression and spatial distribution of cells and ECM substances (Branski et al., 2006; Thibeault et al., 2003; Titze et al., 2004; Verdolini et al., 2003).

The injury mechanism of phonatory stresses to the vocal fold tissue is not yet scientifically proven. However, speculation has arisen due to physical models of vocal fold vibration that describe the magnitude and distribution of the phonatory stresses in the tissue (Gunter, 2003, 2004; Jiang et al., 1998). A three-dimensional finite element model of vocal fold vibration predicted an increase in both impact and vertical shear stresses at the center of the vocal fold edge during vocal fold collision (Gunter, 2003, 2004). This vocal fold location is exactly the injury-prone site where phonotraumatic lesions normally develop. The vocal folds are believed to undergo repetitive microtrauma owing to phonation throughout life. A postmortem study of 266 adult autopsies reported that 36.5% of the vocal folds were considered as normal while 64% presented with microscopic vocal fold lesions (Salge et al., 2006). None of the autopsy cases exhibited clinically significant phonotraumatic lesions. These data suggest that the vocal folds can generally sustain phonatory injury and do not necessarily develop a macroscopic vocal fold lesion throughout life. The vocal folds may be structurally capable of withstanding phonatory stresses and/or may have reparative capabilities to resolve microscopic phonotraumatic damage. However, when the injury culminates in a threshold episode, inflammation becomes evident and may eventually develop macroscopic vocal fold lesions. Phonotrauma can result from a single traumatic force of relatively large magnitude or from repeated forces of relatively small magnitude. When a single vocal loading (e.g. screaming at a football game) produces traumatic injury to vocal fold tissue, the injury is known as *acute phonotrauma*. When repeated or chronic vocal loadings over a period of time produce an injury, the injury is known as *chronic phonotrauma*. Vocal fold nodules, polyps, cysts (sub-epithelial and ligament) and Reinke's edema are the benign vocal fold lesions, owing to chronic phonotrauma.

## Vocal fold scarring

According to the Classification Manual for Voice Disorders-I (CMVD-I; Verdolini et al., 2006: 56), a vocal fold scar is defined as 'a permanent change to the microarchitecture of the lamina propria, consisting of a loss of the viscoelastic properties of the tissue'. Vocal fold scarring can be induced by inflammation or more commonly follows micro-phonosurgery of vocal fold lesions (Hirano, 2005). Numerous studies employ animal models to characterize the histological changes in both acute and chronic vocal fold scarring from surgical trauma.

A vocal fold scar is regarded as a fibrous tissue resulting from a complete wound healing process (Hirano, 2005; Thibeault, 2005). An animal vocal fold scar is characterized by fibrosis (an increase in collagen or procollagen during the early stages of healing) or a disorganized collagen scaffolding (a loss of the regular three-dimensional collagen structure at the end of healing) (Thibeault, 2005). Also, numerous ECM components are altered during vocal fold scarring as seen in animals. Specifically, decreased elastin, increased fibronectin, decreased decorin and decreased fibromodulin are reported, although variations across animal species are noted (Thibeault, 2005). This alteration of the fibrous and interstitial proteins affects the vocal fold cover-body relationship and the propagation of a normal mucosal wave, which severely affects one's voice quality (Thibeault, 2005).

The translation from animal findings to human is a challenge. The difference in the vocal fold architecture and the amount of vocal use between animals and humans is acknowledged in the literature (Benninger et al., 1996). Further, another major concern of using an animal surgical model to mimic the situation in humans following phonosurgery is that the initial state of the vocal fold tissue is fundamentally different between these two models. In current animal models, the surgical procedure is done on healthy and non-scarred vocal fold tissue, whereas in humans the surgical procedure is done on pre-inflamed or pathologic vocal fold tissues. An alternative animal protocol on using pre-inflamed or pre-injured vocal folds is suggested to approximate the scarring process following phonosurgery in humans.

## Contemporary Treatment Approaches for Phonotrauma

Scientific evidence generally supports the idea that targeting voice production work (with or without a so-called indirect therapy or 'vocal hygiene' component) can be effective for a spectrum of voice disorders (Bassiouny, 1998; Chen et al., 2007; Gillivan-Murphy et al., 2006; Kotby et al., 1991; MacKenzie et al., 2001; Rattenbury et al., 2004; Roy et al., 2001, 2003; Sellars et al., 2002; Simberg et al., 2006; Speyer et al., 2002, 2003, 2004a, 2004b; Wingate et al., 2006). Evidence is clearest for some specific benign vocal fold pathologies in particular, namely, contact granuloma and nodules (Behrman et al., 2008; Holmberg et al., 2001; McCrory, 2001; Murry & Woodson, 1992; Verdolini-Marston et al., 1995; Ylitalo & Hammarberg, 2000). However, the investigation of the biological mechanisms underlying the healing effect of voice therapy remains to be explored.

At the time of this writing, no experimental studies have been done on the understanding of the biological effects of tissue mobilization for *chronic* phonotrauma. Only two experimental studies to date have examined the effects of tissue mobilization for *acute* vocal fold inflammation (Branski *et al.*, 2007; Verdolini *et al.*, under review). The first study used an *in vitro* model to evaluate the effects of cyclic equibiaxial tensile strain (CTS) on rabbit vocal fold fibroblast cultures in the presence or absence of interleukin-1β-induced (IL-1β) inflammation (Branski *et al.*, 2007). IL-1β is a key pro-inflammatory cytokine and induces numerous pro-inflammatory mediators, such as inducible nitric oxide synthase (iNOS), nitric oxide (NO), cyclooxygenase-2 (COX-2), prostaglandin E2 (PGE2) and matrix metalloproteases (MMPs). Excessive synthesis of pro-inflammatory markers generally leads to unfavorable healing outcomes (Dinarello, 1997, 2000; Guirao & Lowry, 1996). In this *in vitro* study, CTS was manipulated in the time domain (4–36 continuous hours), in the magnitude domain (0–18%) and in the frequency domain (static–0.5 Hz) in rabbit vocal fold fibroblast cultures in the presence or absence of IL-1β. Results showed that, when the fibroblast cultures were pre-inflamed with IL-1β and stimulated with CTS for 4 hours, iNOS mRNA expression was reduced most under a specific CTS regimen: low magnitude (6%) and relatively high frequency (0.5 Hz). This CTS regimen was then used in two subsequent experiments. The first experiment tested the effects of CTS on the synthesis of COX-2, MMP-1, $PGE_2$ and NO in the fibroblast cultures. Results showed that low magnitude of CTS blocked COX-2, MMP-1 and $PGE_2$ synthesis up to 24 hours and NO up to 36 hours in the IL-1β-induced inflamed cultures, compared to the absence of CTS condition. The second experiment tested the effects of CTS on the synthesis of matrix proteins, namely, procollagen type I IL-1β, which is known to inhibit the synthesis of procollagen type I as, for example, in dermal fibroblasts (Mauviel *et al.*, 1991), lung fibroblasts (Diaz *et al.*, 1993) and osteoblastic cells (Harrison *et al.*, 1990). Counterintuitively, the results from these two experiments showed that CTS upregulated procollagen type I synthesis after 24 or 48 hours of CTS exposure in the IL-1β-induced inflamed vocal fold fibroblast cultures.

The second study investigated the biological effects of voice rest versus two different forms of tissue mobilization (resonant voice exercises and spontaneous speech) for experimentally induced acute vocal fold inflammation in human subjects (Verdolini *et al.*, under review). The main obstacle for this line of research, initially, was the lack of a technology to quantify vocal fold inflammation in human subjects. Recently, a laboratory at the University of Pittsburgh developed an approach that addresses the relevant technological gap. That approach indicated that vocal fold inflammatory and healing states could be evaluated by biochemically assaying vocal fold surface secretions (Sandulache *et al.*, 2007). Preliminary data indicated a correspondence between inflammatory mediator concentrations in secretions and those in tissue in the rabbit subglottis, albeit with a relatively small lag in time and magnitude. Other human surgical data are currently under analysis (Rosen *et al.*, unpublished data). Pending the outcome of those analyses, existing evidence increases confidence in the ability of mediator concentrations in laryngeal secretions to reasonably quantitatively reflect concentrations in tissue. At that level, a methodology has become available to pursue the novel hypothesis that certain forms of tissue mobilization may have value for the modulation of inflammatory and healing states in human vocal folds.

Voice rest, resonant voice exercises and spontaneous speech can be considered on a continuum of tissue mobilization and especially vocal fold impact stress magnitude: (1) none (voice rest), (2) normal- to large-amplitude vocal fold oscillations and low impact stress (resonant voice exercises), and (3) normal- to large-amplitude oscillations but potentially larger impact stress, depending on the speaker (spontaneous speech). Specifically, compared to pressed and breathy phonation modes, resonant voice involves comparatively large-amplitude but low-impact vocal fold vibrations (Berry *et al.*, 2001; Peterson *et al.*, 1994; Verdolini, 2000; Verdolini *et al.*, 1998). The vocal fold vibratory characteristics associated with spontaneous speech vary, but are thought to tend towards pressed speech in many speakers. In the study by Verdolini *et al.* (1998), nine vocally healthy human participants were subjected to a vocal loading task involving 45 minutes of loud voice phonation (75–90 dB SPL at 15 cm microphone-to-mouth distance) during a 1-hour period. Then the participants were randomly assigned to one of three treatment groups: voice rest, resonant voice exercises or spontaneous speech as monitored for 4 hours in the clinic. After a 4-hour treatment period, participants were discharged to home with instructions to continue to follow their corresponding treatment condition. Laryngeal secretions were sampled from the vocal fold surfaces at the following time points: pre-loading (baseline); immediately post-loading; 4 hours post-treatment onset; and 24 hours post baseline. Enzyme-linked immunosorbent assays (ELISA) were then run to measure the concentrations of a panel of biomarkers in the secretions.

Biomarkers concentration results showed that the concentrations of pro-inflammatory mediators (IL-1β, IL-6 and MMP-8) were lowest following resonant voice exercises and highest following the spontaneous speech condition at the 24-hour post baseline time point. At the same time, the concentration of the anti-inflammatory marker IL-10 showed an opposite trend at the 24-hour time point, that is concentrations for this marker were highest following resonant voice exercises and lowest following voice rest. These preliminary findings suggest that large-amplitude, low-impact vocal fold tissue mobilization, as reported for resonant voice exercises, may relatively optimize the quality of the healing response for acute phonotrauma by attenuating pro-inflammatory and stimulating anti-inflammatory responses.

# Contemporary Treatment Approaches for Vocal Fold Scarring

Vocal fold scarring remains one of the most challenging, recalcitrant and functionally debilitating conditions to treat among the conditions affecting voice (Benninger et al., 1996; Hirano, 2005; Rosen, 2000). Tissue engineering approaches utilizing cells and scaffolds have been the two biomimetic approaches for the optimization of vocal fold healing following surgical injury (Kanemaru et al., 2003). The principle is that the scaffold will facilitate the delivery and attachment of injected cells to the defective tissue. Ultimately, the scaffold will be assimilated to become part of the native tissue, whereas the injected cells will secrete a cocktail of mediators and matrices to accelerate healing and restore the defective tissue.

## Scaffolds

Acellular matrix (Chan et al., 2009; Ringel et al., 2006; Xu et al., 2007, 2009), collagen hydrogels (Hahn et al., 2006) and hyaluronic acid (HA)-based hydrogels (Duflo et al., 2006a, 2006b; Finck & Lefebvre, 2005; Finck et al., 2010; Hansen et al., 2005; Hertegard et al., 2006b; Jia et al., 2006; Johnson et al., 2010; Thibeault et al., 2010) have been used for scaffold design in vocal fold scarring. Most studies focused on using HA to develop the scaffold for vocal folds. Because the half-life of native HA is short (Ward et al., 2002), synthetic HA such as Carbylan-GSX has been developed to control HA's turnover rate through crosslinking and chemical modification. Rabbit models have shown that HA-based scaffold decreased fibrosis and improved vocal fold viscoelasticity (Finck & Lefebvre, 2005; Finck et al., 2010; Hertegard et al., 2006b). Further, HA-based scaffold was found to enhance the expression of inflammatory mediators and ECM markers during the acute inflammatory phase, resulting improved tissue composition and viscoelasticity properties of the treated vocal folds at 6 months following surgical injury (Duflo et al., 2006a; Thibeault et al., 2010).

## Cells

Cell-based therapy involves the transplantation of cells into defective tissue to restore functional tissue. Mesenchymal stem cells (MSCs), which are derived from bone marrow, adipose tissue and vocal folds, have been reported to prevent or treat vocal fold scarring, in the absence or presence of scaffolds and regulator factors (Chhetri et al., 2004; Hertegard et al., 2006a, 2006b; Hong et al., 2011; Johnson et al., 2010; Kanemaru et al., 2003, 2005; Kumai et al., 2010; Lee et al., 2006; Ohno et al., 2011; Svensson et al., 2010; Xu et al., 2011).

MSCs are multipotent cells and can differentiate into various lineages, namely chondrocytes, osteoblasts and adipocytes, in vitro and in vivo

(Deans & Moseley, 2000; Pittenger et al., 1999; Tuan et al., 2003; Woodbury et al., 2000). Kanemaru et al. (2003, 2005) used MSCs from bone marrow for transplantation and 1% hydrogen chloride atelocollagen gel as a scaffold to sustain the cells. After injecting the cells into previously injured vocal folds of canine and rat, the vocal fold regeneration was assessed both morphologically and histologically. Injected vocal folds showed normalized macroscopic appearance after 2 months in contrast to imperfect healing (e.g. atrophy, granuloma formation) found in untreated control vocal folds (Kanemaru et al., 2003). A later study by the same group of investigators showed that the MSCs survived and differentiated into at least two laryngeal cell types (epithelial and muscle) in the implanted rat vocal folds (Kanemaru et al., 2005). The researchers suggested that their MSCs produced associated ECM products necessary for healing. Besides the active research of using MSCs for vocal fold regeneration in the USA, Dr Hertegard's laboratory in Sweden (Hertegard et al., 2006a; Svensson et al., 2010) also assessed the regeneration process as a function of viscoelastic and histologic parameters for scarred rabbit vocal folds after the injection of human MSCs. Rabbits were treated with low-dose immunosuppressive drugs. Results showed improved viscoelastic properties (decreased dynamic viscosity and lower elastic modulus) and less signs of scarring (less collagen content) in the implanted vocal folds when compared to the untreated scarred group, up to 3 months following injury. Most recently, Thibeault's laboratory (Johnson et al., 2010) in the USA reported that a combined approach of using bone marrow MSC and HA-based scaffold had better healing outcomes in injured rat vocal folds compared to using bone marrow MSC alone. The foregoing results regarding MSC intervention in traumatized vocal folds are encouraging.

Previous research efforts had focused on how MSCs would differentiate into functional cell types for tissue regeneration (see reviews by Bianco et al., 2008; Kolf et al. 2007; Pittenger et al., 1999). Current opinion, however, is that the main mechanism of MSC-mediated regenerative effects is linked to the cells' immunomodulatory functions rather than to their ability to differentiate into lost cell types (Caplan & Dennis, 2006; van Poll et al., 2008). Both animal and human models suggest that postnatal MSCs have the ability to modulate inflammation and fibrosis to enhance the healing of injured tissue without scarring (Abarbanell et al., 2009; Caplan & Dennis, 2006; Deans & Moseley, 2000; Djouad et al., 2003; Guo et al., 2007; Iyer & Rojas, 2008; Le Blanc et al., 2003; Nauta & Fibbe, 2007; Oh et al., 2008; Ortiz et al., 2003; Pittenger et al., 1999; Rasmusson, 2006; Ren et al., 2008; Togel et al., 2005; Tse et al., 2003; Tuan et al., 2003; Uccelli et al., 2006; van Poll et al., 2008; Yoo et al., 2009). Specifically, MSCs were shown to release a range of cytokines, chemokines, proteases and growth factors to directly modify the healing process in damaged tissue through paracrine mechanisms (Abarbanell et al., 2009; Burchfield & Dimmeler, 2008; Caplan & Dennis, 2006; Crisostomo et al., 2007; Gnecchi et al., 2008; Kumai et al., 2009; Li et al., 2009;

Nauta & Fibbe, 2007; Oh *et al.*, 2009; Rasmusson, 2006; Uccelli *et al.*, 2006; van Poll *et al.*, 2008).

So far, only one study (Kumai *et al.*, 2009) investigated the immuno-modulatory properties of adult stem cells in the context of the vocal folds. Kumai and colleagues co-cultured adipose-derived stem cells with fibro-blasts harvested from scarred ferret vocal folds. Compared to normal fibro-blasts, the scarred fibroblasts proliferated faster, producing less HA but more collagen at Day 7 after culturing. When adipose-derived stem cells and scarred fibroblasts were co-cultured, results showed slower scarred fibro-blast proliferation, and less collagen but similar HA production compared to the monoculture of scarred fibroblasts. Scarred vocal folds following vocal fold 'stripping' is commonly characterized by excessive collagen accumula-tion but diminished HA content in different animal models (Hansen & Thibeault, 2006).

The results from the co-culture study suggested that adipose-derived stem cells may exert *anti-fibrotic* effects on wound vocal fold fibroblasts, which may ultimately promote scarless healing following surgical vocal fold trauma. However, the *anti-inflammatory* effects of adult stem cells have not been studied in the setting of vocal folds. Possible anti-inflammatory func-tions of MSCs include suppression of the immune cell proliferation (dendritic cells, natural killer cells, T-cells and B-cells) (Aggarwal & Pittenger, 2005; Corcione *et al.*, 2006; Jiang *et al.*, 2005; Krampera *et al.*, 2007; Le Blanc, 2006; Maccario *et al.*, 2005; Nauta & Fibbe, 2007; Nauta *et al.*, 2006; Ramasamy *et al.*, 2007; Rasmusson, 2006; Rasmusson *et al.*, 2003; Spaggiari *et al.*, 2008; van Poll *et al.*, 2008) as well as attenuation of pro-inflammatory cytokines (IL-1$\beta$, IL-6, interferon-gamma [IFN-$\gamma$] and tumor necrosis factor [TNF]-$\alpha$) but amplification of anti-inflammatory cytokine (IL-10) expressions in the cases of animal myocardial infarct, lung injury or inflammatory bowel dis-eases (Caplan & Dennis, 2006; Guo *et al.*, 2007; Gupta *et al.*, 2007; Iyer & Rojas, 2008; Nauta & Fibbe, 2007; Panes & Salas, 2009; Rasmusson, 2006; Rojas *et al.*, 2005; van Poll *et al.*, 2008). In fact, inflammation and fibrosis are closely linked. Unresolved inflammation is a major risk factor for fibrosis and scar formation (Diegelmann & Evans, 2004; Hart, 2002; Hunt *et al.*, 2000; Steed, 2003; van Poll *et al.*, 2008). An optimal control of inflammation is the key to tissue regeneration. Further research on the MSC's anti-inflammatory functions in scarred vocal folds is warranted.

Research has been surging to understand the biological response of vocal fold tissue to phonotrauma and voice treatments. Also, contemporary management of vocal fold scarring has been geared towards a tissue-engineering approach, such as the use of cells and scaffolds to treat inflam-mation and optimize the healing of surgically injured vocal folds. The more biological processes are revealed, the clearer will be the understanding of vocal fold health and disease. Very recently, a computational approach has also been applied to integrate the massive biological data and simulate the individual wound healing responses to both acute phonotrauma and surgical vocal fold injury. This new research direction will ultimately accelerate the design of a more individualized, targeted and effective therapy for patients with voice diseases.

## References

Abarbanell, A.M., Coffey, A.C., Fehrenbacher, J.W., Beckman, D.J., Herrmann, J.L., Weil, B., *et al.* (2009) Proinflammatory cytokine effects on mesenchymal stem cell therapy for the ischemic heart. *Annals of Thoracic Surgery* 88 (3), 1036–1043.

Aggarwal, S. and Pittenger, M.F. (2005) Human mesenchymal stem cells modulate allogeneic immune cell responses. *Blood* 105 (4), 1815–1822.

Bassiouny, S. (1998) Efficacy of the accent method of voice therapy. *Folia Phoniatrica et Logopaedica* 50 (3), 146–164.

Behrman, A., Rutledge, J., Hembree, A. and Sheridan, S. (2008) Vocal hygiene education, voice production therapy, and the role of patient adherence: A treatment effectiveness study in women with phonotrauma. *Journal of Speech, Language, and Hearing Research* 51 (2), 350–366.

Benninger, M.S., Alessi, D., Archer, S., Bastian, R., Ford, C., Koufman, J., *et al.* (1996) Vocal fold scarring: Current concepts and management. *Otolaryngology – Head and Neck Surgery* 115 (5), 474–482.

Berry, D.A., Verdolini, K., Montequin, D.W., Hess, M.M., Chan, R.W. and Titze, I.R. (2001) A quantitative output–cost ratio in voice production. *Journal of Speech, Language, and Hearing Research* 44 (1), 29–37.

Bianco, P., Robey, P.G. and Simmons, P.J. (2008) Mesenchymal stem cells: Revisiting history, concepts, and assays. *Cell Stem Cell* 2 (4), 313–319.

Branski, R.C., Verdolini, K., Sandulache, V., Rosen, C.A. and Hebda, P.A. (2006) Vocal fold wound healing: A review for clinicians. *Journal of Voice* 20 (3), 432–442.

Branski, R.C., Perera, P., Verdolini, K., Rosen, C.A., Hebda, P.A. and Agarwal, S. (2007) Dynamic biomechanical strain inhibits IL-1beta-induced inflammation in vocal fold fibroblasts. *Journal of Voice* 21 (6), 651–660.

Burchfield, J.S. and Dimmeler, S. (2008) Role of paracrine factors in stem and progenitor cell mediated cardiac repair and tissue fibrosis. *Fibrogenesis & Tissue Repair* 1 (1), 4.

Calvin, M. (1998) Cutaneous wound repair. *Wounds* 10 (1), 12–32.

Caplan, A.I. and Dennis, J.E. (2006) Mesenchymal stem cells as trophic mediators. *Journal of Cellular Biochemistry* 98 (5), 1076–1084.

Chan, R.W., Rodriguez, M.L. and McFetridge, P.S. (2009) The human umbilical vein with Wharton's jelly as an allogeneic, acellular construct for vocal fold restoration. *Tissue Engineering Part A* 15 (11), 3537–3546.

Chen, S.H., Hsiao, T.Y., Hsiao, L.C., Chung, Y.M. and Chiang, S.C. (2007) Outcome of resonant voice therapy for female teachers with voice disorders: Perceptual, physiological, acoustic, aerodynamic, and functional measurements. *Journal of Voice* 21 (4), 415–425.

Chhetri, D.K., Head, C., Revazova, E., Hart, S., Bhuta, S. and Berke, G.S. (2004) Lamina propria replacement therapy with cultured autologouos fibroblasts for vocal fold scars. *Otolaryngology – Head and Neck Surgery* 131 (6), 864–870.

Corcione, A., Benvenuto, F., Ferretti, E., Giunti, D., Cappiello, V., Cazzanti, F., *et al.* (2006) Human mesenchymal stem cells modulate B-cell functions. *Blood* 107 (1), 367–372.

Crisostomo, P.R., Wang, M., Markel, T.A., Lahm, T., Abarbanell, A.M., Herrmann, J.L., *et al.* (2007) Stem cell mechanisms and paracrine effects: Potential in cardiac surgery. *Shock* 28 (4), 375–383.

Deans, R.J. and Moseley, A.B. (2000) Mesenchymal stem cells: Biology and potential clinical uses. *Experimental Hematology* 28 (8), 875–884.

Diaz, A., Munoz, E., Johnston, R., Korn, J.H. and Jimenez, S.A. (1993) Regulation of human lung fibroblast alpha 1 (I) procollagen gene expression by tumor necrosis factor alpha, interleukin-1 beta, and prostaglandin E2. *Journal of Biological Chemistry* 268 (14), 10364–10371.

Diegelmann, R.F. and Evans, M.C. (2004) Wound healing: An overview of acute, fibrotic and delayed healing. *Frontiers in Bioscience* 9, 283–289.

Dinarello, C.A. (1997) Interleukin-1. *Cytokine & Growth Factor Reviews* 8 (4), 253–265.

Dinarello, C.A. (2000) Proinflammatory cytokines. *Chest* 118 (2), 503–508.

Djouad, F., Pience, P. and Bony, C. (2003) Immunosuppressive effect of mesenchymal stem cells favors tumor growth in allogeneic animals. *Blood* 102, 2837–3844.

Duflo, S., Thibeault, S.L., Li, W., Shu, X.Z. and Prestwich, G. (2006a) Effect of a synthetic extracellular matrix on vocal fold lamina propria gene expression in early wound healing. *Tissue Engineering* 12 (11), 3201–3207.

Duflo, S., Thibeault, S.L., Li, W., Shu, X.Z. and Prestwich, G.D. (2006b) Vocal fold tissue repair *in vivo* using a synthetic extracellular matrix. *Tissue Engineering* 12 (8), 2171–2180.

Finck, C. and Lefebvre, P. (2005) Implantation of esterified hyaluronic acid in microdissected Reinke's space after vocal fold microsurgery: First clinical experiences. *Laryngoscope* 115 (10), 1841–1847.

Finck, C.L., Harmegnies, B., Remacle, A. and Lefebvre, P. (2010) Implantation of esterified hyaluronic acid in microdissected Reinke's space after vocal fold microsurgery: Short- and long-term results. *Journal of Voice* 24 (5), 626–635.

Gillivan-Murphy, P., Drinnan, M.J., O'Dwyer, T.P., Ridha, H. and Carding, P. (2006) The effectiveness of a voice treatment approach for teachers with self-reported voice problems. *Journal of Voice* 20 (3), 423–431.

Gnecchi, M., Zhang, Z., Ni, A. and Dzau, V.J. (2008) Paracrine mechanisms in adult stem cell signaling and therapy. *Circulation Research* 103 (11), 1204–1219.

Gray, S.D. (2000) Cellular physiology of the vocal folds. In C.A. Rosen and T. Murry (eds) *The Otolaryngologic Clinics of North America*. Philadelphia: W.B. Saunders.

Gray, S.D. and Titze, I.R. (1988) Histologic investigation of hyperphonated canine vocal cords. *Annals of Otology, Rhinology and Laryngology* 97 (4), 381–388.

Gray, S.D., Titze, I.R. and Lusk, R.P. (1987) Electron microscopy of hyperphonated canine vocal cords. *Journal of Voice* 1 (1), 109–115.

Gray, S.D., Hirano, M. and Sato, K. (1993) Molecular and cellular structure of vocal fold tissue. In I.R. Titze (ed.) *Vocal Fold Physiology*. San Diego: Singular Publishing.

Gray, S.D., Pignatari, S.S. and Harding, P. (1994) Morphologic ultrastructure of anchoring fibers in normal vocal fold basement membrane zone. *Journal of Voice* 8 (1), 48–52.

Gray, S.D., Titze, I.R., Alipour, F. and Hammond, T.H. (2000) Biomechanical and histologic observations of vocal fold fibrous proteins. *Annals of Otology, Rhinology and Laryngology* 109, 77–85.

Guirao, X. and Lowry, S.F. (1996) Biologic control of injury and inflammation: Much more than too little or too late. *World Journal of Surgery* 20, 437–446.

Gunter, H.E. (2003) A mechanical model of vocal-fold collision with high spatial and temporal resolution. *Journal of the Acoustical Society of America* 113 (2), 994–1000.

Gunter, H.E. (2004) Modeling mechanical stresses as a factor in the etiology of benign vocal fold lesions. *Journal of Biomechanics* 37 (7), 1119–1124.

Guo, J., Lin, G.S., Bao, C.Y., Hu, Z.M. and Hu, M.Y. (2007) Anti-inflammation role for mesenchymal stem cells transplantation in myocardial infarction. *Inflammation* 30 (3–4), 97–104.

Gupta, N., Su, X., Popov, B., Lee, J.W., Serikov, V. and Matthay, M.A. (2007) Intrapulmonary delivery of bone marrow-derived mesenchymal stem cells improves survival and attenuates endotoxin-induced acute lung injury in mice. *Journal of Immunology* 179 (3), 1855–1863.

Hahn, M.S., Teply, B.A., Stevens, M.M., Zeitels, S.M. and Langer, R. (2006) Collagen composite hydrogels for vocal fold lamina propria restoration. *Biomaterials* 27 (7), 1104–1109.

Hansen, J.K. and Thibeault, S.L. (2006) Current understanding and review of the literature: Vocal fold scarring. *Journal of Voice* 20 (1), 110–120.

Hansen, J.K., Thibeault, S.L., Walsh, J.F., Shu, X.Z. and Prestwich, G.D. (2005) *In vivo* engineering of the vocal fold extracellular matrix with injectable hyaluronic acid hydrogels: Early effects on tissue repair and biomechanics in a rabbit model. *Annals of Otology, Rhinology and Laryngology* 114 (9), 662–670.

Hardy, M.A. (1989) The biology of scar formation. *Physical Therapy* 69 (12), 1014–1024.

Harrison, J.R., Vargas, S.J., Petersen, D.N., Lorenzo, J.A. and Kream, B.E. (1990) Interleukin-1 alpha and phorbol ester inhibit collagen synthesis in osteoblastic MC3T3-E1 cells by a transcriptional mechanism. *Molecular Endocrinology* 4 (2), 184–190.

Hart, J. (2002) Inflammation. 2: Its role in the healing of chronic wounds. *Journal of Wound Care* 11 (7), 245–249.

Hertegard, S., Cedervall, J., Svensson, B., Forsberg, K., Maurer, F.H.J., Vidovska, D., *et al.* (2006a) Viscoelastic and histologic properties in scarred rabbit vocal folds after mesenchymal stem cell injection. *Laryngoscope* 116 (1248–1254).

Hertegard, S., Dahlqvist, A. and Goodyer, E. (2006b) Viscoelastic measurements after vocal fold scarring in rabbits – short-term results after hyaluronan injection. *Acta Oto-laryngologica* 126 (7), 758–763.

Hirano, M. (1977) Structure and vibratory behavior of the vocal folds. In M. Sawashima and S.C. Fankin (eds) *Dynamic Aspects of Speech Production* (pp. 13–30). Tokyo: University of Tokyo Press.

Hirano, M. (1981) Structure of the vocal fold in normal and disease states: Anatomical and physical studies. Paper presented at the Assessement of Vocal Pathology, Rockville.

Hirano, M. and Kakita, Y. (1985) Cover-body theory of vocal fold vibration. In R.G. Daniloff (ed.) *Speech Science*. San Diego: College-Hill Press.

Hirano, M. and Sato, K. (1993) *Histological Color Atlas of the Human Larynx*. San Diego: Singular Publishing.

Hirano, M., Kurita, S. and Nakashima, T. (1981) The structure of the vocal folds. In K.N. Stevens and M. Hirano (eds) *Vocal Fold Physiology*. Tokyo: University of Tokyo Press.

Hirano, S. (2005) Current treatment of vocal fold scarring. *Current Opinion in Otolaryngology & Head and Neck Surgery* 13 (3), 143–147.

Holmberg, E.B., Hillman, R.E., Hammarberg, B., Sodersten, M. and Doyle, P. (2001) Efficacy of a behaviorally based voice therapy protocol for vocal nodules. *Journal of Voice* 15 (3), 395–412.

Hong, S.J., Lee, S.H., Jin, S.M., Kwon, S.Y., Jung, K.Y., Kim, M.K., *et al.* (2011) Vocal fold wound healing after injection of human adipose-derived stem cells in a rabbit model. *Acta Oto-laryngologica* 131 (11), 1198–1204.

Hunt, T.K., Hopf, H. and Hussain, Z. (2000) Physiology of wound healing. *Advances in Skin & Wound Care* 13 (Suppl. 2), 6–11.

Iyer, S.S. and Rojas, M. (2008) Anti-inflammatory effects of mesenchymal stem cells: Novel concept for future therapies. *Expert Opinion on Biological Therapy* 8 (5), 569–581.

Jia, X., Yeo, Y., Clifton, R.J., Jiao, T., Kohane, D.S., Kobler, J.B., *et al.* (2006) Hyaluronic acid-based microgels and microgel networks for vocal fold regeneration. *Biomacromolecules* 7 (12), 3336–3344.

Jiang, J.J., Diaz, C.E. and Hanson, D.G. (1998) Finite element modeling of vocal fold vibration in normal phonation and hyperfunctional dysphonia: Implications for the pathogenesis of vocal nodules. *Annals of Otology, Rhinology and Laryngology* 107, 603–610.

Jiang, X.X., Zhang, Y., Liu, B., Zhang, S.X., Wu, Y., Yu, X.D., *et al.* (2005) Human mesenchymal stem cells inhibit differentiation and function of monocyte-derived dendritic cells. *Blood* 105 (10), 4120–4126.

Johnson, B.Q., Fox, R., Chen, X. and Thibeault, S. (2010) Tissue regeneration of the vocal fold using bone marrow mesenchymal stem cells and synthetic extracellular matrix injections in rats. *Laryngoscope* 120 (3), 537–545.

Kanemaru, S., Nakamura, T., Omori, K., Kojima, H., Magrufov, A., Hiratsuka, Y., *et al.* (2003) Regeneration of the vocal fold using autologous mesenchymal stem cells. *Annals of Otology, Rhinology and Laryngology* 112 (11), 915–920.

Kanemaru, S., Nakamura, T., Yamashita, M., Magrufov, A., Kita, T., Tamaki, H., *et al.* (2005) Destiny of autologous bone marrow-derived stromal cells implanted in the vocal fold. *Annals of Otology, Rhinology and Laryngology* 114 (12), 907–912.

Kolf, C.M., Cho, E. and Tuan, R.S. (2007) Mesenchymal stromal cells. Biology of adult mesenchymal stem cells: Regulation of niche, self-renewal and differentiation. *Arthritis Research & Therapy* 9 (1), 204.

Kotby, M.N., El-Sady, S.R., Basiouny, S.E., Abou-Rass, Y.A. and Hegazi, M.A. (1991) Efficacy of the accent method of voice therapy. *Journal of Voice* 5, 316–320.

Krampera, M., Sartoris, S., Liotta, F., Pasini, A., Angeli, R., Cosmi, L., *et al.* (2007) Immune regulation by mesenchymal stem cells derived from adult spleen and thymus. *Stem Cells and Development* 16 (5), 797–810.

Kumai, Y., Kobler, J.B., Park, H., Lopez-Guerra, G., Karajanagi, S., Herrera, V.L., *et al.* (2009) Crosstalk between adipose-derived stem/stromal cells and vocal fold fibroblasts *in vitro. Laryngoscope* 119 (4), 799–805.

Kumai, Y., Kobler, J.B., Herrera, V.L. and Zeitels, S.M. (2010) Perspectives on adipose-derived stem/stromal cells as potential treatment for scarred vocal folds: Opportunity and challenges (Review). *Current Stem Cell Research & Therapy* 5 (2), 175–181.

Le Blanc, K. (2006) Mesenchymal stromal cells: Tissue repair and immune modulation. *Cytotherapy* 8 (6), 559–561.

Le Blanc, K., Tammki, L., Sundberg, B., Haynesworth, S.E. and Ringden, O. (2003) Mesenchymal stem cells inhibit and stimulate mixed lymphocyte cultures and mitogenic response independently of the major histocompatibility complex. *Scandinavian Journal of Immunology* 57, 11–20.

Lee, B.J., Wang, S.G., Lee, J.C., Jung, J.S., Bae, Y.C., Jeong, H.J., *et al.* (2006) The prevention of vocal fold scarring using autologous adipose tissue-derived stromal cells. *Cells Tissues Organs* 184 (3–4), 198–204.

Li, L., Zhang, S., Zhang, Y., Yu, B., Xu, Y. and Guan, Z. (2009) Paracrine action mediate the antifibrotic effect of transplanted mesenchymal stem cells in a rat model of global heart failure. *Molecular Biology Reports* 36 (4), 725–731.

Maccario, R., Podesta, M., Moretta, A., Cometa, A., Comoli, P., Montagna, D., *et al.* (2005) Interaction of human mesenchymal stem cells with cells involved in alloantigen-specific immune response favors the differentiation of CD4+ T-cell subsets expressing a regulatory/suppressive phenotype. *Haematologica* 90 (4), 516–525.

MacKenzie, K., Millar, A., Wilson, J.A., Sellars, C. and Deary, I.J. (2001) Is voice therapy an effective treatment for dysphonia? A randomised controlled study. *British Medical Journal* 323, 1–6.

Mast, B.A. (1992) The skin. In I.K. Cohen, B. Diegelmann and W.J. Lindblad (eds) *Wound Healing: Biochemical and Clinical Aspects.* Philadelphia: W.B. Saunders.

Mauviel, A., Heino, J., Kahari, V.M., Hartmann, D.J., Loyau, G., Pujol, J.P., *et al.* (1991) Comparative effects of interleukin-1 and tumor necrosis factor-alpha on collagen production and corresponding procollagen mRNA levels in human dermal fibroblasts. *Journal of Investigative Dermatology* 96 (2), 243–249.

McCrory, E. (2001) Voice therapy outcomes in vocal fold nodules: A retrospective audit. *International Journal of Langguage & Communucation Disorders* Suppl. 36, 19–24.

Murry, T. and Woodson, G.E. (1992) A comparison of three methods for the management of vocal fold nodules. *Journal of Voice* 6 (3), 271–276.

Nauta, A.J. and Fibbe, W.E. (2007) Immunomodulatory properties of mesenchymal stromal cells. *Blood* 110 (10), 3499–3506.

Nauta, A.J., Kruisselbrink, A.B., Lurvink, E., Willemze, R. and Fibbe, W.E. (2006) Mesenchymal stem cells inhibit generation and function of both CD34+-derived and monocyte-derived dendritic cells. *Journal of Immunology* 177 (4), 2080–2087.

Oh, J.Y., Kim, M.K., Shin, M.S., Lee, H.J., Ko, J.H., Wee, W.R., *et al.* (2008) The anti-inflammatory and anti-angiogenic role of mesenchymal stem cells in corneal wound healing following chemical injury. *Stem Cells* 26 (4), 1047–1055.

Oh, J.Y., Kim, M.K., Shin, M.S., Wee, W.R. and Lee, J.H. (2009) Cytokine secretion by human mesenchymal stem cells cocultured with damaged corneal epithelial cells. *Cytokine* 46 (1), 100–103.

Ohno, S., Hirano, S., Kanemaru, S., Kitani, Y., Kojima, T., Tateya, I., *et al.* (2011) Implantation of an atelocollagen sponge with autologous bone marrow-derived mesenchymal stromal cells for treatment of vocal fold scarring in a canine model. (Research support, non-US Gov). *Annals of Otology, Rhinology and Laryngology* 120 (6), 401–408.

Ortiz, L.A., Gambelli, F. and McBride, C. (2003) Mesenchymal stem cell engraftment in lung is enhanced in response to bleomycin exposure and ameliorates its fibrotic effects. *Proceedings of the National Academy of Science* 100, 8407–8411.

Panes, J. and Salas, A. (2009) Mechanisms underlying the beneficial effects of stem cell therapies for inflammatory bowel diseases. *Gut* 58 (7), 898–900.

Peterson, K.L., Verdolini-Marston, K., Barkmeir, J.M. and Hoffman, H.T. (1994) Comparison of aerodynamic and electroglottographic parameters in evaluating clinically relevant voicing patterns. *Annals of Otology, Rhinology and Laryngology* 103 (5, Part 1), 335–346.

Pittenger, M.F., Mackay, A.M., Beck, S.C., Jaiswal, R.K., Douglas, R., Mosca, J.D., *et al.* (1999) Multilineage potential of adult human mesenchymal stem cells. *Science* 284 (5411), 143–147.

Ramasamy, R., Fazekasova, H., Lam, E.W., Soeiro, I., Lombardi, G. and Dazzi, F. (2007) Mesenchymal stem cells inhibit dendritic cell differentiation and function by preventing entry into the cell cycle. *Transplantation* 83 (1), 71–76.

Rasmusson, I. (2006) Immune modulation by mesenchymal stem cells. *Experimental Cell Research* 312 (12), 2169–2179.

Rasmusson, I., Ringden, O., Sundberg, B. and Le Blanc, K. (2003) Mesenchymal stem cells inhibit the formation of cytotoxic T lymphocytes, but not activated cytotoxic T lymphocytes or natural killer cells. *Transplantation* 76 (8), 1208–1213.

Rattenbury, H.J., Carding, P.N. and Finn, P. (2004) Evaluating the effectiveness and efficiency of voice therapy using transnasal flexible laryngoscopy: A randomized controlled trial. *Journal of Voice* 18 (4), 522–533.

Ren, G., Zhang, L., Zhao, X., Xu, G., Zhang, Y., Roberts, A.I., *et al.* (2008) Mesenchymal stem cell-mediated immunosuppression occurs via concerted action of chemokines and nitric oxide. *Cell Stem Cell* 2 (2), 141–150.

Ringel, R.L., Kahane, J.C., Hillsamer, P.J., Lee, A.S. and Badylak, S.F. (2006) The application of tissue engineering procedures to repair the larynx. *Journal of Speech, Language, and Hearing Research* 49 (1), 194–208.

Rojas, M., Xu, J., Woods, C.R., Mora, A.L., Spears, W., Roman, J., *et al.* (2005) Bone marrow-derived mesenchymal stem cells in repair of the injured lung. *American Journal of Respiratory Cell and Molecular Biology* 33 (2), 145–152.

Rosen, C.A. (2000) Vocal fold scar. In C.A. Rosen and T. Murry (eds) *The Otolaryngologica Clinics of North America. Voice Disorders and Phonosurgery*. Philadelphia: W.B. Saunders.

Rosen, C.A., Li, N.Y.K., Hebda, P.A. and Verdolini, K. Correspondence of inflammatory mediators in laryngeal secretions and laryngeal tissue (unpublished data).

Roy, N., Gray, S.D., Simon, M., Dove, H., Corbin-Lewis, K. and Stemple, J.C. (2001) An evaluation of the effects of two treatment approaches for teachers with voice disorders:

A prospective randomized clinical trial. *Journal of Speech, Language, and Hearing Research* 44, 286–296.

Roy, N., Weinrich, B., Gray, S.D., Tanner, K., Stemple, J.C. and Sapienza, C.M. (2003) Three treatments for teachers with voice disorders: A randomized clinical trial. *Journal of Speech, Language, and Hearing Research* 46 (3), 670–688.

Salge, A.K., Peres, L.C., Reis, M.A., Teixeira Vde, P. and Castro, E.C. (2006) Histopathologic changes in human true vocal folds: A postmortem study. *Annals of Diagnostic Pathology* 10 (5), 274–278.

Sandulache, V.C., Chafin, J.B., Li-Korotky, H.S., Otteson, T.D., Dohar, J.E. and Hebda, P.A. (2007) Elucidating the role of interleukin 1beta and prostaglandin E2 in upper airway mucosal wound healing. *Archives of Otolaryngology – Head & Neck Surgery* 133 (4), 365–374.

Santoro, M.M. and Gaudino, G. (2005) Cellular and molecular facets of keratinocyte reepithelization during wound healing. *Experimental Cell Research* 304 (1), 274–286.

Sellars, C., Carding, P.N., Deary, I.J., MacKenzie, K. and Wilson, J.A. (2002) Characterization of effective primary voice therapy for dysphonia. *Journal of Laryngology & Otology* 116, 1014–1018.

Simberg, S., Sala, E., Tuomainen, J., Sellman, J. and Ronnemaa, A.M. (2006) The effectiveness of group therapy for students with mild voice disorders: A controlled clinical trial. *Journal of Voice* 20 (1), 97–109.

Spaggiari, G.M., Capobianco, A., Abdelrazik, H., Becchetti, F., Mingari, M.C. and Moretta, L. (2008) Mesenchymal stem cells inhibit natural killer-cell proliferation, cytotoxicity, and cytokine production: Role of indoleamine 2,3-dioxygenase and prostaglandin E2. *Blood* 111 (3), 1327–1333.

Speyer, R., Weinke, G., Hosseini, E.G., Kempen, E.G., Kersing, W. and Dejonckere, P.H. (2002) Effects of voice therapy as objectively evaluated by digitized laryngeal stroboscopic imaging. *Annals of Otology, Rhinology and Laryngology* 111 (10), 902–908.

Speyer, R., Wieneke, G.H., van Wijck-Warnaar, I. and Dejonckere, P.H. (2003) Effects of voice therapy on the voice range profiles of dysphonic patients. *Journal of Voice* 17 (4), 544–556.

Speyer, R., Wieneke, G.H. and Dejonckere, P.H. (2004a) Documentation of progress in voice therapy: Perceptual, acoustic, and laryngostroboscopic findings pretherapy and posttherapy. *Journal of Voice* 18 (3), 325–340.

Speyer, R., Wieneke, G.H. and Dejonckere, P.H. (2004b) Self-assessment of voice therapy for chronic dysphonia. *Clinical Otolaryngology and Allied Sciences* 29 (1), 66–74.

Stadelmann, W.K., Digenis, A.G. and Tobin, G.R. (1998) Physiology and healing dynamics of chronic cutaneous wounds. *American Journal of Surgery* 176 (Suppl. 2A), 26S–38S.

Steed, D.L. (2003) Wound-healing trajectories. *Surgical Clinics of North America* 83 (3), 547–555, vi–vii.

Svensson, B., Nagubothu, R.S., Cedervall, J., Le Blanc, K., Ahrlund-Richter, L., Tolf, A., *et al.* (2010) Injection of human mesenchymal stem cells improves healing of scarred vocal folds: Analysis using a xenograft model. *Laryngoscope* 120 (7), 1370–1375.

Thibeault, S.L. (2005) Advances in our understanding of the Reinke space. *Current Opinion in Otolaryngology & Head and Neck Surgery* 13, 148–151.

Thibeault, S.L., Hirschi, S.D. and Gray, S.D. (2003) DNA microarray gene expression analysis of a vocal fold polyp and granuloma. *Journal of Speech, Language, and Hearing Research* 46 (2), 491–502.

Thibeault, S.L., Klemuk, S.A., Chen, X. and Quinchia Johnson, B.H. (2010) In vivo engineering of the vocal fold ECM with injectable HA hydrogels – late effects on tissue repair and biomechanics in a rabbit model. *Journal of Voice* 25 (2), 249–253.

Titze, I.R. (1989) On the relation between subglottal pressure and fundamental frequency in phonation. *Journal of the Acoustical Society of America* 85, 901–906.

Titze, I.R., Hitchcock, R.W., Broadhead, K., Webb, K., Li, W., Gray, S.D., *et al.* (2004) Design and validation of a bioreactor for engineering vocal fold tissues under combined tensile and vibrational stresses. *Journal of Biomechanics* 37 (10), 1521–1529.

Titze, I.R., Hunter, E.J. and Svec, J.G. (2007) Voicing and silence periods in daily and weekly vocalizations of teachers. *Journal of the Acoustical Society of America,* 121 (1), 469–478.

Togel, F., Hu, Z., Weiss, K., Isaac, J., Lange, C. and Westenfelder, C. (2005) Administered mesenchymal stem cells protect against ischemic acute renal failure through differentiation-independent mechanisms. *American Journal of Physiology – Renal Physiology* 289 (1), F31–42.

Tse, W.T., Pendleton, J.D., Beyer, W.M., Egalka, M.C. and Guinan, E.C. (2003) Suppression of allogeneic T-cell proliferation by human marrow stromal cells: Implications in transplantation. *Transplantation* 75 (3), 389–397.

Tuan, R.S., Boland, G. and Tuli, R. (2003) Adult mesenchymal stem cells and cell-based tissue engineering. *Arthritis Research & Therapy* 5 (1), 32–45.

Uccelli, A., Moretta, L. and Pistoia, V. (2006) Immunoregulatory function of mesenchymal stem cells. *European Journal of Immunology* 36 (10), 2566–2573.

van Poll, D., Parekkadan, B., Borel Rinkes, I.H.M., Tilles, A.W. and Yarmush, M.L. (2008) Mesenchymal stem cell therapy for protection and repair of injured vital organs. *Cellular and Molecular Bioengineering* 1 (1), 42–59.

Verdolini, K. (2000) Resonant voice therapy. In J.C. Stemple (ed.) *Voice Therapy: Clinical Studies* (pp. 46–62). San Deigo: Singular Publishing.

Verdolini, K., Druker, D.G., Palmer, P.M. and Samawi, H. (1998) Laryngeal adduction in resonant voice. *Journal of Voice* 12 (3), 315–327.

Verdolini, K., Rosen, C.A., Branski, R.C. and Hebda, P.A. (2003) Shifts in biochemical markers associated with wound healing in laryngeal secretions following phonotrauma: A preliminary study. *Annals of Otology, Rhinology, & Laryngology* 112 (12), 1021–1025.

Verdolini, K., Rosen, C.A. and Branski, R.C. (2006) *Classification Manual for Voice Disorders – I.* New Jersey: Lawrence Erlbaum.

Verdolini, K., Li, N.Y.K., Branski, R.C., Rosen, C.A., Urban, E.G. and Hebda, P.A. (under review) The effect of targeted vocal exercise on recovery from acute inflammation.

Verdolini-Marston, K., Burke, M.K., Lessac, A., Glaze, L. and Caldwell, E. (1995) Preliminary study of two methods of treatment for laryngeal nodules. *Journal of Voice* 9 (1), 74–85.

Ward, P.D., Thiebault, S.L. and Gray, S.D. (2002) Hyaluronic acid: Its role in voice. *Journal of Voice* 16 (3), 303–309.

Wingate, J.M., Brown, W.S., Shrivastav, R., Davenport, P. and Sapienza, C.M. (2006) Treatment outcomes for professional voice users. *Journal of Voice* 21 (4), 433–449.

Witte, M.B. and Barbul, A. (1997) General principles of wound healing. *Surgical Clinics of North America* 77 (3), 509–528.

Woodbury, D., Schwarz, E.J., Prockop, D.J. and Black, I.B. (2000) Adult rat and human bone marrow stromal cells differentiate into neurons. *Journal of Neuroscience Research* 61 (4), 364–370.

Xu, C.C., Chan, R.W. and Tirunagari, N. (2007) A biodegradable, acellular xenogeneic scaffold for regeneration of the vocal fold lamina propria. *Tissue Engineering* 13 (3), 551–566.

Xu, C.C., Chan, R.W., Weinberger, D.G., Efune, G. and Pawlowski, K.S. (2009) A bovine acellular scaffold for vocal fold reconstruction in a rat model. *Journal of Biomedical Materials Research Part A* 92 (1), 18–32.

Xu, W., Hu, R., Fan, E. and Han, D. (2011) Adipose-derived mesenchymal stem cells in collagen-hyaluronic acid gel composite scaffolds for vocal fold regeneration (Research support, non-US Gov). *Annals of Otology, Rhinology and Laryngology* 120 (2), 123–130.

Ylitalo, R. and Hammarberg, B. (2000) Voice characteristics, effects of voice therapy, and long-term follow-up of contact granuloma patients. *Journal of Voice* 14 (4), 557–566.

Yoo, K.H., Jang, I.K., Lee, M.W., Kim, H.E., Yang, M.S., Eom, Y., *et al.* (2009) Comparison of immunomodulatory properties of mesenchymal stem cells derived from adult human tissues. *Cellular Immunology* 259 (2), 150–156.

# 12  Cognitive Behavioural Therapy in the Treatment of Functional Dysphonia in the United Kingdom

## Paul Carding, Vincent Deary and Tracy Miller

This chapter describes the rationale and preliminary evidence for the use of cognitive behavioural therapy (CBT) techniques in the treatment of patients with functional dysphonia (FD). The first section defines the relevant terms and concepts. The second section describes a preliminary effectiveness study which aimed to produce pilot data as to the possible benefit of using CBT techniques in the treatment of FD. The third section provides a broad discussion of the major issues surrounding this programme and how one may continue to investigate the value of this approach.

## Defining the Terms and Concepts

### Functional dysphonia

It is clear that there is considerable confusion and controversy over the nomenclature and classification of voice disorders. This is perhaps most succinctly articulated by Baker *et al.* in a recent review which lists at least 13 common terminologies for the non-organic voice disorders (Baker *et al.*, 2007). Functional dysphonia is a term which is commonly used to describe voice problems where there is no organic cause for the disorder. It can (or at least should) therefore be seen as distinct from organic voice disorders (where the dysphonia is due to mass lesions, structural changes or neurological impairment). However it should be noted that 'functional' also has connotations which are peculiar to the voice field. For example, some authors use the term to specifically refer to disorders that are exclusively secondary to vocal cord misuse, while others use it as synonymous with psychogenic (Greene & Mathieson, 2001). For the purposes of this chapter, our use of the term 'functional dysphonia' is closest to Baker's definition (Baker et al., 2007), where it is used to cover all instances of voice production problems where there is no obvious lesion or injury to the vocal folds, or where the degree of lesion or injury is not sufficient to account for the impairment.

These types of voice disorder represent the most common presentation to many voice clinics (Carding, 2003). Patients with FD have been shown to have increased levels of psychological distress, poorer quality of life and more medically unexplained symptoms than normal controls (White et al., 1997; Wilson et al., 2002).

## Conventional treatment for FD

The treatment of choice for patients with FD is specialist speech/voice therapy. Most treatment programmes involve a combination of 'direct' treatment techniques (such as specific vocal function exercises) and 'indirect' techniques (such as vocal hygiene advice, vocal education and non-directive counselling) (Carding, 2000; Carding et al., 1999). The principle aim of these intervention strategies is to restore normal voice quality and normal laryngeal phonatory behaviour and appearance. There is good quality, robust evidence for the effectiveness of these conventional speech/voice therapy treatment programmes (e.g. Carding, 2000; Carding et al., 1999; MacKenzie et al., 2001; Ruotsalainen et al., 2007). These studies all show significant improvement from baseline using outcome measures of perceptual voice quality ratings, voice handicap scores and sound-signal acoustic analysis. A recent systematic review (Ruotsalainen et al., 2007) has correctly highlighted the shortcomings in our evidence base. Nevertheless, the methodological quality of the published studies has resulted in the reasonable conclusion that these voice improvements are due to the therapy administered (as opposed to any other major influencing factor).

## Psychological well-being and FD

A number of studies (e.g. Deary et al., 1997; MacKenzie et al., 2001; White et al., 1997) have shown that patients with FD have high levels of psychological distress and that this is a major factor in their poor quality of life ratings. However, present evidence suggests that conventional voice therapy approaches do not have a significant effect on these areas. For example, by far the largest randomised controlled trial of voice therapy effectiveness ($N = 133$) showed that conventional voice therapy significantly improved voice quality and voice handicap but that the associated levels of anxiety, depression and poor general health remained virtually unchanged in this patient population (MacKenzie et al., 2001). In fact, in most voice therapy effectiveness studies these psychological factors have not been measured or targeted in treatment at all.

## Cognitive behavioural therapy

Cognitive behavioural psychology offers a theoretically coherent model of why symptoms arise in the absence of organic pathology. This model in turn suggests treatment strategies and has proved acceptable to patients as a treatment rationale.

The cognitive behavioural model distinguishes between the developmental predispositions and precipitants which start a problem and the cognitive, behavioural, affective and physiological factors that interact to perpetuate it (Allen *et al.*, 2002; Beck, 1976). The generic hypothesis is that predisposing and precipitating factors (such as personality traits, childhood adversity, stressful life events and viruses) serve to trigger an initial period of physical symptoms. These are then maintained by an interplay of factors. For instance, a combination of chronic habituation, increased symptom focus, catastrophic interpretation of symptoms, avoidance behaviour and low mood may become locked into a self-maintaining cycle. CBT tends to focus initially on this perpetuating cycle, attempting to dismantle the interlock of factors hypothesised to perpetuate the symptoms (see, for instance, Hutton, 2005; Richardson & Engel, 2004; Surawy *et al.*, 1995 in other related disorders).

## CBT and FD

It is clear that a multifactorial model of FD fits well with the cognitive-behavioural model described above. Previous authors have also written about these conceptual models of non-organic dysphonia (Butcher *et al.*, 1987). In UK practice, it is also clear that speech and language therapists already use a variety of psychology-based interventions, but in an ad hoc fashion with few attempts to identify their clinical effectiveness (separate from that of the specific voice techniques). These observations would suggest that UK speech and language therapists may be a suitable and appropriate group of professionals to deliver (additional) CBT interventions to dysphonic patients. It would appear reasonable to treat these areas of psychological distress alongside trying to improve voice quality. This may result in a more holistic rehabilitation for the patient and reduce the chances of remission and/or transference onto other medically unexplained symptoms. However, there is not as yet any specific evidence to support adopting this approach.

# Developing an Evidence Base

Because of the lack of evidence, a pragmatic pilot study was conducted to investigate the additional benefit of 'Cognitive Behavioural Therapy enhanced voice therapy' in the treatment of patients with FD. For practical and methodological reasons (explained below), a consecutive cohort design was used. The first group of functional dysphonic patients ($N = 16$) were treated with conventional voice therapy (defined below) by one specialist voice therapist. The therapist was then trained in CBT theory and practice (defined below). A second cohort of patients ($N = 16$) were then treated with CBT-enhanced voice therapy (defined below) by the same therapist. Measures of voice, general health and psychological well-being were taken pre- and post-treatment (defined below). It was hypothesised that both groups of patients would improve on measures of voice quality and voice handicap. It was also hypothesised that the CBT-enhanced voice therapy would improve general health and psychological distress more than those who received conventional voice therapy alone.

## Patients

All patients were examined using endoscopy and stroboscopy and were diagnosed as having FD (i.e. dysphonia in the absence of a structural lesion or vocal cord movement disorder). Patients were excluded from the study if:

(1)  they had undergone previous voice therapy, phonosurgery or CBT;
(2)  they declined voice therapy; or
(3)  their condition did not warrant a full course of voice therapy, that is if they had minimal vocal dysfunction (as judged by the clinician's GRBAS rating) or minimal vocal handicap (as measured by the patient's completion of the Vocal Performance Questionnaire).

## Treatment

All patients (i.e. both treatment cohorts) were given six sessions of voice therapy once a week (this represents an average length of a course of voice therapy in the UK; Dunnet *et al.*, 1997). All speech therapy sessions lasted approximately 60 minutes to minimise the inter-group difference in total contact time with the therapist. All patients in the study (i.e. both treatment cohorts) were treated by the same expert voice therapist.

### Conventional voice therapy

Voice therapy sessions followed a conventional format of direct and indirect treatment strategies as previously described in the literature (Carding, 2000; Carding *et al.*, 1999; MacKenzie *et al.*, 2001). Indirect therapy included aspects such as vocal hygiene advice, voice conservation and general relaxation techniques. Direct therapy included techniques to modify vocal behaviour such as airflow techniques, laryngeal deconstruction therapy, pitch modification and reduction of hard glottal attack. The aim of therapy was to restore the patient's voice to normal functioning levels (for that individual). Of the 16 patients in this cohort, all completed treatment but one did not complete outcome data.

*CBT training*

The expert voice clinician was then trained in the principles and practice of CTB. The trainer was a cognitive behavioural therapist specialising in the treatment of medically unexplained symptoms. The training consisted of an initial intensive 5-day training programme with two 1-day follow-up sessions. The training focussed on the following areas:

(1) Understanding the CBT theoretical model of medically unexplained symptoms and how this model may pertain to our understanding of the cause and treatment of FD.
(2) Teaching practical assessment techniques to help identify the predisposing and perpetuating factors which may underpin the voice disorder.
(3) Formulating and delivering a treatment rationale based on the assessment findings.
(4) Using specific techniques aimed at the identified maintaining factors of the voice disorder.

*CBT-enhanced voice therapy*

The voice clinician then delivered the CBT-enhanced voice therapy to a second cohort of 16 patients. Therapy timescales and contact time were kept the same as for the conventional therapy group – six weekly 1-hour sessions. The CBT intervention was delivered in conjunction with conventional voice therapy techniques (as described above). In general, the CBT part of the therapy programme involved three different elements: (1) identifying maintaining factors for the voice disorder; (2) brief behavioural interventions of relevant areas (principally activity/rest management and gradual exposure to avoidances); and (3) identifying and challenging negative thinking patterns. The ongoing supervision by the CBT trainer during the second treatment phase was 1 hour weekly for the first 3 months, then fortnightly or as requested. More details about the CBT treatments can be found in Appendix 12.A at the end of this chapter.

Three patients dropped out of this treatment arm, one at session 2 and the other two at session 4. No outcome data was collected from them.

## Outcome measures

Treatment outcome measures of voice, general health and psychological well-being were taken before and after treatment. It was hypothesised that both treatment groups would perform equally well on the voice outcome measures (GRBAS Ratings of Voice Quality, Voice Performance Questionnaire (VPQ) and Voice Symptoms Scale (VoiSS), described below) but that the CBT group would show greater improvement on the general health and psychology well-being measures (Hospital Anxiety and Depression scale (HAD) and General Health Questionnaire (GHQ-28), described below).

### GRBAS ratings of voice quality

Voice samples were recorded using high quality digital facilities following a standard protocol (Carding, 2000). Each voice was rated using the GRBAS rating scale (Hirano, 1981) by an independent therapist using a randomly ordered set of samples. The GRBAS scale requires an expert listener to rate one 'overall severity' grade and four defining aspects of voice quality (roughness, breathiness, asthenia and strain) using a 0–3 scale (0 = normal; 3 = severely abnormal). In all cases the rater was blinded to the treatment group and status of the patients. The GRBAS scale has been shown to be a reliable and robust clinical measure of voice quality, with an intra-rater reliability of overall severity of 0.81 and an inter-rater reliability of 0.78, as measured by intra-class correlation (Webb *et al.*, 2004). In our study the same judge re-rated 20% of the voices 1 month later in order to calculate intra-rater reliability.

### Voice Performance Questionnaire (VPQ)

The VPQ is a 12-item single trait self-report measure of the patient's voice performance and utility. It has proved reliable and sensitive as an indicator of how the subject has been affected by the voice disorder during daily normal functioning. Each item is scored on a 5-point scale from 1 (no adverse effect) to 5 (severe effect). Hence a total severity score could range from 12 (normal) to 60 (severely abnormal) (Carding, 2000; Carding *et al.*, 1999; Deary *et al.*, 2004).

### The Voice Symptoms Scale (VoiSS)

The VoiSS is a psychometrically robust measurement of the importance and severity of a patient's voice-related symptoms. It is a 30-question self-report scale which gives an overall numerical score with a minimum of 0 and a maximum of 120, indicating the overall level of voice disorder. It comprises three sub-scales, evaluating Impairment, Emotional and Physical factors (Deary *et al.*, 2003).

### The Hospital Anxiety and Depression scale (HAD)

The HAD (Zigmond & Snaith, 1983) is a widely used self-rated measure of psychological distress. It has two subscales of seven questions each, measuring anxiety and depression, each with a score range of 0 to 21. Clinically significant levels of anxiety and depression are generally regarded to be of a score of 8 or more on either sub-scale (Goldberg *et al.*, 1997). A previous randomised controlled trial (MacKenzie *et al.*, 2001) showed that the HAD was not responsive to change following conventional voice therapy.

### The General Health Questionnaire-28 (GHQ)

The GHQ-28 (Goldberg & Williams, 1988) is a measure of general well-being and distress. It has also been shown to be sensitive to change in a variety of trials for medically unexplained symptoms (Kroenke & Swindle, 2000). The GHQ-28 has 28 items, comprising seven questions in four sub-scales of anxiety and insomnia, somatisation, depression and social dysfunction. Questions have four possible responses, from 'no problem' to 'severe', and can be scored either scaled (0011) or Likert (0123). We chose the latter as more sensitive to clinical change. Scored thus, clinically significant levels of well-being and distress have a threshold of 23 or above (Goldberg *et al.*, 1997).

## Data analysis

### Assessment of baseline differences in study groups

Student's unpaired *t*-test was used to assess the groups for baseline differences. Clearly, major differences at baseline would have a bearing on how differences post-treatment should be interpreted.

### Assessment of treatment outcomes in study groups

Using the paired *t*-test, pre- and post-treatment mean values for all outcome measures were compared for the control (conventional voice therapy) and experimental (CBT-enhanced voice therapy) groups separately. Student's unpaired *t*-test was then used to compare the mean change due to treatment for the control and CBT groups. All available data were entered into the final analysis, that is 15 from the control group and 13 from the CBT group.

### Assessment of effect sizes in study groups

Within-group effect sizes were estimated by subtracting the mean score at baseline from the mean score at outcome and dividing by the standard deviation (S.D.) of control group at baseline. Between-group effect sizes were calculated by dividing mean difference in outcome by baseline standard deviation of control group.

## Results

### Assessment of baseline differences in study groups

There were no significant between-group differences at baseline in the voice measures (see Tables 12.1 and 12.2). There was a trend for the CBT group to be more distressed at baseline. Although none of these differences was significant, the CBT group did approach the threshold of 8 for anxiety on the HAD and were over the Likert threshold (cut-off 23/24) in the GHQ-28. However, given the small sample size and non-significance of these differences, it was considered not meaningful to control for them in the final analyses.

### Assessment of treatment outcomes in study groups

Both groups improve significantly on both self-rated quality of voice measures. Only the CBT group improves significantly on objectively rated voice quality (GRBAS). There is a trend towards significance in the between-group difference in this measure. Both groups improved significantly on the GHQ total score, with the CBT group improving significantly more than the controls.

**Table 12.1** Mean and standard deviation (S.D.) of the outcome measures of both subject groups

| | VoiSS | VPQ | GRBAS | GHQ | HAD Anxiety | HAD Depression |
|---|---|---|---|---|---|---|
| Controls (N = 15) | 51.6 ± 18.6 | 38.4 ± 8.3 | 1.7 ± 1.3 | 20.3 ± 8.6 | 5.3 ± 4.0 | 3.2 ± 3.3 |
| CBT (N = 13) | 58.3 ± 18.2 | 36.6 ± 8.6 | 1.9 ± 1.0 | 27.9 ± 14.2 | 7.9 ± 4.1 | 5.6 ± 3.8 |
| Mean dif. | 6.7 | −1.8 | 0.2 | 7.7 | 2.6 | 2.4 |
| 95% Cl | −7.6 to 21.0 | −8.3 to 4.8 | −0.7 to 1.1 | −1.6 to 16.9 | −0.6 to 5.7 | −0.4 to 5.2 |
| P value | 0.345 | 0.580 | 0.673 | 0.091 | 0.103 | 0.084 |

Notes: Statistics given are: mean ± S.D., lower and upper 95% confidence intervals.
VoiSS, Voice Symptoms Scale; VPQ, Voice Performance Questionnaire; GHQ, General Health Questionnaire; HAD, Hospital Anxiety and Depression scale; CBT, Cognitive Behavioural Therapy subject group.

The CBT group scores improved significantly in HAD depression while the control group's HAD scores hardly changed at all. This between-group difference showed a trend towards significance in HAD depression scores. In terms of clinical significance, the mean scores for HAD anxiety and GHQ total fell below the thresholds following treatment in the CBT group. The most notable results are illustrated in Figures 12.1 and 12.2.

## Assessment of effect sizes in study groups

Finally, the within-group effect sizes were greater for CBT on all measures. Voice therapy alone had no effect on either HAD score. The relative effect size of CBT-enhanced voice therapy compared to conventional voice therapy alone was greatest for GHQ (1.4) and HAD depression (0.8), with a trend towards a significant effect size for GRBAS (0.6).

Both groups improve significantly on both self-rated quality of voice measures. Only the CBT group improve significantly on objectively rated voice quality (GRBAS). There is a trend towards significance in the between-group difference in this measure. Both groups improved significantly on the GHQ total score, with the CBT group improving significantly more than the controls.

The CBT group scores improved significantly in HAD depression and almost significantly in HAD anxiety while the control groups' HAD scores hardly changed at all. This between-group difference showed a trend towards significance in HAD depression scores. In terms of clinical significance, the mean scores for HAD anxiety and GHQ total fell below the thresholds following treatment in the CBT group. The most notable results are illustrated in Figures 12.1 and 12.2.

**Table 12.2** Differences within groups following treatment, and between-group differences post treatment

|  | VoiSS total | VPQ total | GRBAS grade | GHQ total | HADS Anxiety | HADS Depression |
|---|---|---|---|---|---|---|
| *Control group (N = 15)* |  |  |  |  |  |  |
| Pre-treatment | 51.6 ± 18.6 | 38.4 ± 8.3 | 1.7 ± 1.3 | 20.3 ± 8.6 | 5.3 ± 4.0 | 3.2 ± 3.3 |
|  | 41.3 to 61.9 | 33.8 to 43.0 | 1.0 to 2.4 | 15.5 to 25.0 | 3.1 to 7.5 | 1.4 to 5.0 |
| Post-treatment | 35.1 ± 19.1 | 26.1 ± 8.7 | 1.1 ± 1.1 | 15.4 ± 7.7 | 5.3 ± 4.2 | 3.1 ± 3.5 |
|  | 24.5 to 45.6 | 21.2 to 30.9 | 0.5 to 1.8 | 11.1 to 19.7 | 3.0 to 7.7 | 1.1 to 5.0 |
| Change pre to post | −16.5 ± 16.2 | −12.3 ± 7.6 | −0.6 ± 1.4 | −4.9 ± 6.2 | 0.0 ± 2.9 | −0.1 ± 2.7 |
| (i.e. outcome) | −25.5 to −7.6 | −16.5 to −8.1 | −1.3 to 0.1 | −8.3 to −1.5 | −1.6 to 1.6 | −1.6 to 1.3 |
| Effect size change ÷ pre-treat S.D. | −0.9 | −1.5 | −0.5 | −0.6 | 0.0 | 0.0 |
| P (pre to post) paired t-test | 0.001* | <0.001* | 0.108 | 0.008* | 1.000 | 0.849 |
| *CBT group (N = 13)* |  |  |  |  |  |  |
| Pre-treatment | 58.3 ± 18.2 | 36.6 ± 8.6 | 1.9 ± 1.0 | 27.9 ± 14.2 | 7.9 ± 4.1 | 5.6 ± 3.8 |
|  | 47.3 to 69.3 | 31.4 to 41.8 | 1.3 to 3.6 | 19.4 to 36.5 | 5.4 to 10.4 | 3.3 to 7.9 |
| Post-treatment | 33.7 ± 19.9 | 23.4 ± 7.8 | 0.5 ± 0.8 | 14.7 ± 7.1 | 6.2 ± 3.3 | 3.2 ± 2.1 |
|  | 21.7 to 45.7 | 18.5 to 28.4 | 0.0 to 0.9 | 10.4 to 19.0 | 4.2 to 8.2 | 0.0 to 0.9 |
| Change pre to post | −24.6 ± 19.9 | −15.0 ± 9.0 | −1.5 ± 1.2 | −13.2 ± 11.6 | −1.7 ± 2.8 | −2.4 ± 3.4 |
| (i.e. outcome) | −36.6 to −12.6 | −20.7 to −9.3 | −2.2 to −0.7 | −20.3 to −6.2 | −3.4 to 0.0 | −4.4 to −0.3 |
| Effect size change ÷ pre-treat S.D. | −1.4 | −1.8 | −1.4 | −0.9 | −0.4 | −0.6 |
| P (pre to post) paired t-test | 0.001* | <0.001* | 0.001* | 0.001* | 0.051 | 0.026* |
| *Difference in outcome (control to CBT)* |  |  |  |  |  |  |
| Difference in outcome (control to CBT) | −8.1 ± 25.6 | −2.7 ± 11.8 | −0.9 ± 1.8 | −8.4 ± 13.2 | −1.7 ± 4.0 | −2.3 ± 4.3 |
|  | −22.3 to 6.1 | −9.4 to 4.0 | −1.9 to 0.1 | −15.7 to −1.0 | −3.9 to 0.5 | −4.6 to 0.1 |
| Effect size difference ÷ control S.D. | −0.5 | −0.4 | −0.6 | −1.4 | −0.6 | −0.8 |
| P (control to CBT) unpaired t-test, eq var | 0.252 | 0.412 | 0.088 | 0.022 | 0.131 | 0.060 |
| Power calc N (power = 0.8, p < 0.05) | 80 | 150 | 33 | 21 | 45 | 29 |

Notes: *Significant at 0.05 level.

Statistics given are: mean ± S.D., lower and upper 95% confidence intervals.

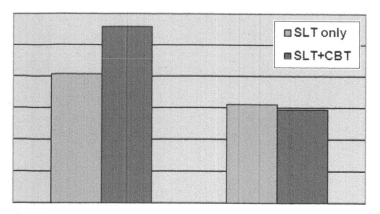

**Figure 12.1** GHQ scores

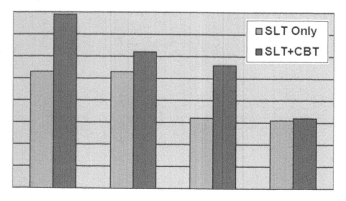

**Figure 12.2** HAD anxiety and depression scores

# Discussion: The Future of CBT and Voice Disorders

## Comments on the preliminary evidence

The preliminary study described above provided some valuable data on a new approach to the treatment of FD. Firstly, traditional voice outcome measures showed significant improvement in both treatment groups. Interestingly, there are some indications that CBT may augment vocal improvement. Secondly, the study shows a significant change in measures of depression and general health only for those patients who received the CBT-enhanced voice therapy. Voice therapy alone had zero effect on HAD scores, and only a modest effect size on GHQ score compared to the CBT group. Putting aside for the moment the between-group baseline differences in these measures, the within-group change in the CBT cohort is both statistically and clinically significant. This indicates that with a brief train-ing it is possible for speech therapists to target the psychological distress, general health and voice quality of dysphonic patients. This 'combined' treatment approach took the same amount of time as conventional voice therapy alone. The only added element, after the brief training, was the supervision by the CBT expert. As the trial proceeded, and the speech/voice therapist became more confident with the CBT intervention, supervision became fortnightly and of shorter duration. This indicates the possibility of significantly improved clinical management of FD with relatively little addi-tional expert input.

These findings corroborate that the transmission of clinically useful CBT skills to non-mental-health professionals is feasible within a relatively short timescale. Other studies, using similar methodologies, have also reported the 'added value' of CBT training to other health care and medical professionals. For example a recent study trained specialist nurses in CBT for irritable bowel syndrome (Kennedy et al., 2005).

## Further development of the evidence base

This preliminary study indicates that the addition of CBT skills to a speech and language therapists may be clinically effective in treating voice quality and psychological distress in FD. Clearly these results cannot be generalised to all speech therapists in all centres. Larger studies will allow us to further assess both the clinical effectiveness of this general approach and the health economics implications, where symptomatic improvement and decreased health care use will need to be balanced against training and supervision costs. Given the brevity of the training and the relatively low supervision input, this pilot tentatively points to a promising future for this work.

There are, however, some considerable limitations to the present study. Firstly, the numbers in both arms of the trial are too small to allow adequate generalisation and definitive conclusions. It should also be noted that there were marked, though non-significant, between-group baseline differences, with the CBT cohort showing a trend towards increased psychological distress and poorer general health. Encouragingly, these respond well to treatment, but it makes between-group comparisons of this effect difficult. There is a possibil-ity in this pilot of a 'floor effect', in that, although the control group do not change on this measure, the CBT group are more distressed pre-treatment so both cohorts end up at a similar level of distress post-treatment. It could be argued that baseline level of distress is the predictor of change in treatment, rather than the treatment itself. However, in the randomised controlled trial by MacKenzie et al. (2001), where distress did not respond to voice therapy alone, the patients had levels of distress similar to the present CBT cohort, suggesting that the CBT arm of the pilot did benefit from a treatment effect. A larger randomised controlled trial with better matched groups would be needed to allow a more definitive conclusion. Re-analysis of our recruitment procedures cannot ascertain a viable reason for these baseline differences. It is likely, given the small numbers, that this is a random effect.

A further potential weakness in the preliminary evidence is the use of a consecutive cohort design, where a single clinician delivered both interventions. While this has the benefit of eliminating inter-therapist variability, it creates the possibility of a time effect, and limits the generalisability of the findings. However, this design does reduce the possibility of a contamination effect, in that the CBT training could not influence the 'pure' voice therapy that preceded it.

Finally, as in many previous studies, this study only reports on outcomes at the immediate post-treatment time point. The longer-term benefits of voice therapy treatment for functional voice disorders are unknown, as are re-occurrence rates. It could be hypothesised that CBT, by targeting not just the symptoms but the factors underlying their maintenance, could reduce re-occurrence of both dysphonia and other medically unexplained symptoms in this group. This type of analysis would, however, involve long-term follow-up and coordination across multiple health service organisations. A more realistic approach would be to analyse FD re-occurrence rates across the two treatment groups.

## CBT and other voice disorders

As Lancaster *et al.* (2004) remind us, the interpretation of pilot work should be mainly descriptive. What the present study illustrated, above all, was that teaching CBT to a speech and language therapist was both feasible and had a positive impact on clinical practice. This has potential implications for the management of other disorders seen by speech and language therapists. Psychogenic aphonia is perhaps the most obvious, where a similar model to that developed in FD could be directly applied. CBT is also being increasingly used to help people adjust to chronic health complaints such as multiple sclerosis (Van Kessel *et al.*, 2008). Similar approaches could therefore be explored in chronic voice disorders such as spasmodic dysphonia, vocal fold paralysis, laryngeal papillomatosis or even in the management of head and neck cancer.

# Conclusion

A recent paper by Baker [30] reviews the research on psychosocial factors in FD and highlights the central importance of addressing these in treatment. Baker, like other authors, notes the lack of consistent training in psychosocial skills for speech and language therapists, but goes further in stating that it is the 'professional and ethical duty' of the profession to acquire and use these skills in treating this disorder. Our pilot work, demonstrated that CBT skills are both easily transmissible and effective in changing UK clinical practice in a way that could potentially benefit not only FD but also other conditions routinely seen by speech and language therapists. This pilot study has also informed the design of a randomised controlled trial of the additional benefit of CBT-enhanced voice therapy for patients with FD.

# References

Allen, L., Escobar, J., Lehrer, P., Gara, M. and Woolfolk, R. (2002) Psychosocial treatments for multiple unexplained physical symptoms: A review of the literature. *Psychosomatic Medicine* 64 (6), 939–950.

Baker, J. (2008) The role of psychogenic and psychosocial factors in the development of functional voice disorders. *International Journal of Speech-Language Pathology* 10, 210–230.

Baker, J., Ben-Tovim, D., Butcher, A., Esterman, A. and McLaughlin, K. (2007) Development of a modified diagnostic classification system for voice disorders with inter-rater reliability study. *Logopedics, Phoniatrics, Vocology* 32 (3), 99–112.

Beck, A. (1976) *Cognitive Therapy and the Emotional Disorders.* New York: Meridian.

Butcher, P., Elias, A., Raven, R., Yeatman, J. and Littlejohns, D. (1987) Psychogenic voice disorder unresponsive to speech therapy: Psychological characteristics and cognitive-behaviour therapy. *British Journal of Disorders of Communication* 22, 81–92.

Carding, P. (2000) *Evaluating Voice Therapy: Measuring the Effectiveness of Treatment.* London: Whurr Publishers.

Carding, P. (2003) Voice pathology in the United Kingdom. *British Medical Journal* 327 (7414), 514–515.

Carding, P., Horsley, I. and Docherty, G. (1999) A study of the effectiveness of voice therapy in the treatment of 45 patients with nonorganic dysphonia. *Journal of Voice* 13 (1), 72–104.

Deary, I., Scott, S. and Wilson, I., *et al.* (1997) Personality and psychological distress in dysphonia. *British Journal of Health Psychology* 2, 1–9.

Deary, I., Wilson, J., Carding, P. and MacKenzie, K. (2003) VoiSS: A patient-derived Voice Symptom Scale. *Journal of Psychosomatic Research* 54 (5), 483–489.

Deary, I., Webb, A., MacKenzie, K., Wilson, J. and Carding, P. (2004) Short, self-report voice symptom scales: Psychometric characteristics of the Voice Handicap Index-10 and the Vocal Performance Questionnaire. *Head & Neck Surgery* 131, 232–235.

Dunnet, C.P., MacKenzie, K., Sellars, G.C., Robinson, K. and Wilson, J.A. (1997) Voice therapy for dysphonia – still more art than science? *European Journal of Disorders of Communication* 32 (3, Special Issue), 333–343.

Goldberg, D. and Williams, P. (1988) *A User's Guide to the General Health Questionnaire.* Windsor: NFER.

Goldberg, D., Gater, R., Sartorius, N., Ustun, T., Piccinelli, M., Gureje, O., *et al.* (1997) The validity of two versions of the GHQ in the WHO study of mental illness in general health care. *Psychological Medicine,* 27 (1), 191–197.

Greene, M.L. and Mathieson, L. (2001) *The Voice and Its Disorders.* London: Whurr Publishers.

Hirano, M. (1981) *Clinical Examination of Voice* (Disorders of Human Communication, No. 5). New York: Springer.

Hutton, J. (2005) Cognitive behaviour therapy for irritable bowel syndrome. *European Journal of Gastroenterology & Hepatology* 17 (1), 11–14.

Kennedy, T., Jones, R., Darnley, S., Seed, P., Wessely, S. and Chalder, T. (2005) Cognitive behaviour therapy in addition to antispasmodic treatment for irritable bowel syndrome in primary care: Randomised controlled trial. *British Medical Journal* 331 (7514), 435.

Kroenke, K. and Swindle, R. (2000) Cognitive-behavioral therapy for somatization and symptom syndromes: A critical review of controlled clinical trials. *Psychotherapy and Psychosomatics* 69 (4), 205–215.

Lancaster, G., Dodd, S. and Williamson, P. (2004) Design and analysis of pilot studies: Recommendations for good practice. *Journal of Evaluation in Clinical Practice* 10 (2), 307–312.

MacKenzie, K., Millar, A., Wilson, J., Sellars, C. and Deary, I. (2001) Is voice therapy an effective treatment for dysphonia? A randomised controlled trial. *British Medical Journal* 323 (7314), 658–661.

Richardson, R. and Engel Jr, C. (2004) Evaluation and management of medically unexplained physical symptoms. *Neurologist* 10 (1), 18–30.

Ruotsalainen, J., Sellman, J., Lehto, L., Jauhiainen, M. and Verbeek, J. (2007) Interventions for treating functional dysphonia in adults. *Cochrane Database of Systematic Reviews* 3 (online).

Surawy, C., Hackmann, A., Hawton, K. and Sharpe, M. (1995) Chronic fatigue syndrome: A cognitive approach. *Behaviour Research and Therapy* 33 (5), 535–544.

Van Kessel, K., Moss-Morris, R., Willoughby, E., Chalder, T., Johnson, M. and Robinson, E. (2008) A randomized controlled trial of cognitive behavior therapy for multiple sclerosis fatigue. *Psychosomatic Medicine* 70 (2), 205–213.

Webb, A., Carding, P., Deary, I., MacKenzie, K., Steen, N. and Wilson, J. (2004) The reliability of three perceptual evaluation scales for dysphonia. *European Archives of Oto-Rhino-Laryngology* 261 (8), 429–434.

White, A., Deary, I. and Wilson, J. (1997) Psychiatric disturbance and personality traits in dysphonic outpatients. *European Journal of Disorders of Communication* 32 (3, Special Issue), 307–314.

Wilson, J., Deary, I., Millar, A. and Mackenzie, K. (2002) The quality of life impact of dysphonia. *Clinical Otolaryngology & Allied Sciences* 27 (3), 179–182.

Zigmond, A. and Snaith, R. (1983) The hospital anxiety and depression scale. *Acta Psychiatrica Scandinavica* 67 (6), 361–370.

# Appendix 12.A The CBT Interventions

Following careful and structured case history taking, the therapist would present to the patient a formulation of their problem that attempted to explain how current factors might be interacting to maintain both poor voice and general distress, and how these had developed through the interaction of predisposing and precipitating factors. So, for example, if the patient was generally fatigued, low in mood, having negative thoughts about activity and so avoiding social and physical activity, and avoiding using their voice (a fairly typical example), it might be suggested that this pattern of general withdrawal and low activity levels were contributing to ongoing low mood, low energy and poor voice, and that working on these factors might help improve things. This formulation then formed the basis for both treatment and treatment supervision.

Treatment was generally a mixture of the following interventions. As each patient had an individualised formulation, no two treatments were the same, but typically consisted of a mixture of the following interventions.

- *Interventions for low energy and low mood.* These were chiefly behavioural, based on the best current evidence. Gradually doing more in a structured planned way and gradually resuming activities that used to be done for enjoyment and achievement are easily taught and transmitted evidence-based interventions for both low mood and low energy. The target behaviours were lack of activity, and the mechanism of change is thought to be both physical re-conditioning (fatigue change) and the re-instituting of regimes of reward and achievement (mood change). This activity management approach also involved some basic sleep management techniques, such as having a bedtime routine and a fixed getting-up time. Again this is thought to target both fatigue and mood, as both tend to involve sleep routine disruption. All of this was planned in session and done as 'homework' by the patient in between sessions.

- *Interventions for anxiety.* As people who are anxious tend to avoid whatever they are anxious of (and thus become more anxious), the main technique used here was again behavioural: encouraging people to gradually confront, at their own pace, difficult situations in a planned and structured way. Avoidance was thus the target behaviour, with increased exposure and desensitisation the proposed mechanism of change. Again, this work was planned in session and done as homework. This often involved simple cognitive techniques, such as helping the patient identify what kind of anxious thoughts they might be having about avoided situations, and helping them to test out the reality of these thoughts by confronting the situation in a safe, planned manner. Cognitive work was thus conceptualised as being an adjunct and an aide to behavioural change.

- *Interventions for unhelpful beliefs.* Some patients in our pilot study had very high self-standards and were very self-critical. The other common unhelpful beliefs were to do with the best way to manage voice and other physical symptoms, with patients often interpreting symptoms as a sign to stop activity altogether and to socially withdraw, thus keeping going a cycle of physical disuse, low energy and low mood. Simple cognitive techniques were identified that would help the patients spot their unhelpful beliefs and test them out by looking for evidence both for and against them. As such beliefs that were maintaining unhelpful behavioural patterns were the targets, insight and challenge were the proposed means of change, and changes in voice and disability measures of avoided/difficult activity were the proposed measures of change. Obviously it is impossible to say whether behaviour change was mediated by prior cognitive change but, pragmatically, these techniques are a common part of CBT treatments and were deemed to be useful by both the supervisor and the speech and language therapist. Again, these techniques were practiced and planned in session and done as homework.

- *Relapse prevention.* Patients were encouraged to practice techniques they found useful, until they could use them independently. At the end of therapy, future difficult situations were anticipated and planned for, and they were encouraged to draw up goals for ongoing work on their vocal and general health improvement. The rationale behind this comes from work that shows anticipation of difficulty and pre-planning coping reduces rate of relapse in some conditions.

Treatment was allowed to take its natural course, in terms of both length and number of sessions (both were monitored and are reported on). Overall, the spirit of the interventions was collaborative and individualised. Nothing was assumed in advance and patients were encouraged to take control of their own treatment. The interventions described were relatively basic and quite simple to execute.

# Introduction to Chapters 13 and 14: Contemporary Voice Research in Hong Kong

Edwin M-L. Yiu

## Introduction

There has been a strong influence of laryngology on the speech therapy service and research in Hong Kong. The speech therapy profession in Hong Kong first started in the early 1960s within the ear, nose and throat (ENT) department in the public hospital setting (Stokes & Yiu, 1997). In 1997, the Voice Research Laboratory was set up under the Division of Speech and Hearing Sciences at the University of Hong Kong (HKU). The Voice Research Laboratory conducts research related to voice science and disorders. The majority of voice research conducted in Hong Kong has been on clinical voice assessment and treatment. A more in-depth review of the different aspects of voice research conducted in Hong Kong can be found in a recent book chapter by Ma and Yiu (2012). Details will not be repeated here, but a brief overview of these areas will be outlined in the next chapter by Yiu (Chapter 13). Chapter 13 also reviews the special development of the application of traditional Chinese medicine in voice treatment. Ma will present another chapter (Chapter 14) with a more in-depth discussion of recent voice motor learning research developed in Hong Kong. These two chapters together represent the two major current areas of voice research in Hong Kong.

## References

Ma, E.P-M. and Yiu, E.M-L. (2012) Voice research in Hong Kong: Past, present and future. In R. Goldfarb (ed.) *Translational Speech Language Pathology & Audiology*. San Diego: Plural Publishing.

Stokes, S.F. and Yiu, E. (1997) Speech therapy and general practice in Hong Kong. *Hong Kong Practitioner* 19 (7), 374–379.

# 13 Acupuncture and Voice Treatment

## Edwin M-L. Yiu

## Overview of Voice Research in Hong Kong Circa 1996–2012

Speech therapy services in Hong Kong have roots going back to the early 1960s, with the first speech therapy service established primarily to address the need for voice therapy (Stokes & Yiu, 1997). Systematic voice research began in 1996 at the University of Hong Kong (HKU) and, a year later, the HKU Voice Research Laboratory was established. The initial research focus covered three very different areas: auditory-perceptual voice evaluation, voice-related quality of life and instrumental voice analysis. These have led to the development of two sets of clinical assessment tools: the auditory-perceptual training protocol for Cantonese voice quality evaluation (Chan & Yiu, 2002, 2006; Yiu et al., 2007), and the Voice Activity and Participation Profile (VAPP; Ma & Yiu, 2001). The VAPP has subsequently been adopted in clinical practice in a number of different languages, which include Brazilian-Portuguese (Ricarte et al., 2006), Croatian (Bonetti et al., 2009), and Finnish (Sukanen et al., 2007).

Research in instrumental voice analysis covered acoustic perturbation analysis (Ma & Yiu, 2005), voice range profile (Ma et al., 2007), aerodynamic measures (Yiu et al., 2004), and high-speed laryngoscopic analysis (Yiu et al., 2010). The findings from these studies allow us to understand better the usefulness and limitations of these different instrumentations used in clinical voice evaluation. Practitioners in Hong Kong and worldwide are now better informed as to when to use these instrumentations and when not to use them.

More recently, voice researchers in Hong Kong have focused more on the treatment or therapy aspect of voice problems. The exploration of alternative treatment methods has extended to the use of traditional Chinese medicine, specifically acupuncture (Yiu et al., 2006). At the same time, the principles of motor learning have begun to be applied in voice therapy in recent years

(Yiu *et al.*, 2005). Voice motor learning research will be described in more detail in the next chapter, while the rest of this chapter will describe the use of acupuncture in treating benign vocal fold lesions.

## Current Traditional Treatment Options for Phonotraumatic Lesions

Conservative behavioural voice therapy is often the first line of treatment for benign vocal pathologies related to phonotrauma (MacKenzie *et al.*, 2001; Ramig & Verdolini, 1998). The surgical option is usually reserved for recalcitrant vocal lesions (Colton *et al.*, 2006; Courey & Ossoff, 2003), and it is not uncommon for phonotraumatic lesions to recur postoperatively. The success of surgery indeed relies heavily on postoperative behavioural voice therapy (Rubin & Yanagisawa, 2003). It has been reported that as high as 20% of the dysphonic population would not benefit from these two treatment options (Woo *et al.*, 1994). In developed countries, there are an increasing number of people seeking alternative non-western treatment (Eisenberg *et al.*, 1993, 1998) with increasing popularity and worldwide acceptance (WHO, 2002). One of the most common alternative or complementary treatment approaches is traditional Chinese medicine. Hong Kong has long been considered a hub for western and eastern cultures. Therefore, studies of traditional Chinese medicine using the western scientific approach have gained much momentum in recent years.

## Acupuncture as an Alternative Treatment Option for Phonotrauma Lesions

Acupuncture has been shown to be effective in treating some types of voice problems (Yang, 2000; Yao, 2000; Yiu *et al.*, 2006). Traditional Chinese medicine views voice problems as being caused by not enough pectoral qi (chest energy/air), an excessive 'yai qi' ('hot air' – excessive heat, i.e. heat and poison), too much phlegm and a 'yin-deficiency' (dehydration). They consider that these conditions cause blockages in the meridians that result in imbalances. The use of acupuncture or acupressure helps to unblock the disruption and maintain a good balance. Needling at specific acupoints is suggested to trigger neurotransmissions that deliver messages to the corresponding cortical areas of the brain (Mann, 1983, 1992). This will then stimulate higher brain centres (e.g. the hypothalamus and amygdala) to issue regulatory instructions to the autonomic nervous system, leading to corresponding healing activities at the disordered organ (Cho *et al.*, 2001).

Yiu *et al.* (2006) reported a randomised prospective study, adopting a standardised acupuncture protocol and using objective quantitative outcome measures as well as quality-of-life outcome measures. In the study, 24 female subjects with either vocal nodules, vocal polyps or vocal fold thickening were randomly assigned to a treatment group that received genuine acupuncture at voice-related acupoints that included Renyin (St9), Lieque (Lu7) and Zhaohai (Ki6), or to a placebo group that received acupuncture at non-voice related acupoints, Houxi (SI3) and Kunlun (Bl60). Both groups received ten 30-minute sessions of acupuncture within a 20-day period. Results showed that genuine acupuncture brought about significantly greater improvements in fundamental frequency functions, breathiness, roughness and VAPP (Ma & Yiu, 2001) scores as compared to the results from the placebo acupuncture.

In order to determine whether acupuncture is merely a placebo effect, a study was carried out to examine the salivary cortisol level in individuals who received genuine or sham acupuncture at acupoints Renyin (St9), Lianquan (Ren23), Lieque (Lu7), Hegu (Li4) and Zhaohai (Ki6) (Kwong & Yiu, 2010). Salivary cortisol has been shown to relate to stress level. For the genuine acupuncture group, the needles used in the acupuncture penetrated the skin surface and entered the acupoints at a pre-defined depth. For the sham acupuncture, the needles did not penetrate the skin but remained on the skin surface of the acupoints. The subjects had no way of telling whether they received the genuine or the sham acupuncture. A high salivary cortisol level indicated relatively higher stress. The study did not show any significant reduction in the cortisol level following the genuine or sham acupuncture. Therefore, the acupuncture effect cannot be attributed to the placebo effect of stress reduction alone (Kwong & Yiu, 2010).

Yiu and colleagues conducted a double-blind randomised control trial with 97 dysphonic subjects using acupuncture. The experimental group ($N = 33$) received genuine acupuncture at acupoints Renyin (St9), Lianquan (Ren23), Lieque (Lu7), Hegu (Li4) and Zhaohai (Ki6), while the sham ($N = 34$) group were made to believe that they also received needles at these acupoints but in reality the needles did not penetrate the skin (Yiu *et al.*, in progress). The deception was achieved by using blunt needles exerting pressure on the skin surface of the acupoints, each of which was covered by a piece of foam board with the needle supported by a plastic catheter (see Figure 13.1). There was also a control group ($N = 30$) with dysphonic subjects who received no acupuncture. The examiners who collected the outcome measures from the subjects were not aware of the type of acupuncture (genuine versus sham) the subjects received. The results on vocal function using a phonetogram, after receiving 12 half-hour sessions of acupuncture over a 6-week period, showed significant improvements in maximum fundamental frequency (see Figure 13.2), auditory-perceptual voice quality and VAPP scores in the experimental (genuine) group.

Interestingly, the data also showed that stimulating the acupoints on the skin surface produced similar effectiveness to the real acupuncture which involved needle penetration beneath the skin at the acupoints.

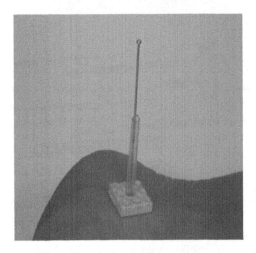

**Figure 13.1** Tubing guide for acupuncture needle

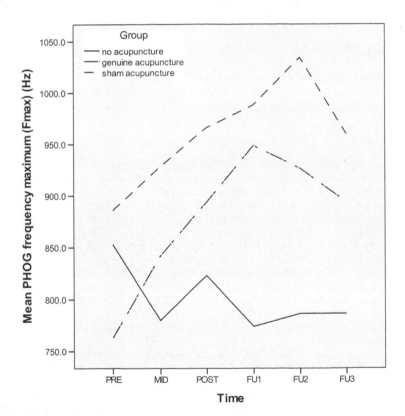

**Figure 13.2** Change of maximum fundamental frequency over time
Notes: PRE, pre-acupuncture; MID, mid-acupuncture; POST, post-acupuncture; FU1, follow-up 1;
FU2, follow-up 2; FU3, follow-up 3.

# Summary

In summary, the studies reviewed above showed that acupuncture with the appropriate acupoints is effective in improving the vocal functions in phonotraumatic voice problems. The effectiveness seemed to be unrelated to a placebo effect as acupuncture of non-related acupoints did not bring about similar improvement. Furthermore, our preliminary data also showed that stimulation of the relevant acupoints even on the skin surface would bring about similar improvement. The underlying mechanism is not clear at this stage, but our preliminary data also found that some biological markers (cytokines) were found to have significantly changed following the acupuncture. This suggested that acupuncture might have facilitated or sped up the wound-healing process. We are also investigating the use of lasers to stimulate the acupoints. Laser stimulation of acupoints has been shown to be effective in treating other types of disorders (Naeser et al., 1995; Radmayr et al., 2001; Wozniak et al., 2003). This non-invasive procedure may be suitable for those individuals who cannot tolerate the needles involved in traditional acupuncture.

## Acknowledgements

The studies reported in this chapter were supported in part by an R21 Grant 5R21AT3879-2 from the National Center for Complementary and Alternative Medicine, National Institute of Health.

## References

Bonetti, A., Simunjak, B. and Bonetti, L. (2009) Samoprocjena I objekivna procjena vokalnih teskoca u osoba s disfonijom. *6th Kongres Hrvatskog drustva za otorinolaringologiju I kirurgiju glave i vrata s medunarodnim* [in Croatian].

Chan, K.M-K. and Yiu, E.M-L. (2002) The effect of anchors and training on the reliability of perceptual voice evaluation. *Journal of Speech, Language, and Hearing Research* 45 (1), 111–126.

Chan, K.M.K. and Yiu, E.M.L. (2006) A comparison of two perceptual voice evaluation training programs for naive listeners. *Journal of Voice* 20 (2), 229–241.

Cho, Z.H., Na, C.S., Wang, E.K., Lee, S.H. and Hong, I.K. (2001) Functional magnetic resonance imaging of the brain in the investigation of acupuncture. In G. Stux and R. Hammerschlag (eds) *Clinical Acupuncture. Scientific Basis* (pp. 83–95). Heidelberg: Springer.

Colton, R.H., Casper, J.K. and Leonard, R. (2006) *Understanding Voice Problems: A Physiological Perspective for Diagnosis and Treatment* (3rd edn). Baltimore: Lippincott Williams & Wilkins.

Courey, M.S. and Ossoff, R.H. (2003) Surgical management of benign voice disorders. In J.S. Rubin, R.T. Sataloff and G.S. Korovin (eds) *Diagnosis and Treatment of Voice Disorders* (2nd edn). New York: Thomson Learning.

Eisenberg, D.M., Kessler, R.C., Foster, C., Norlock, F.E., Calkins, D.R. and Delbanco, T.L. (1993) Unconventional medicine in the United States. Prevalence, costs, and patterns of use. *New England Journal of Medicine* 328 (4), 246–252.

Eisenberg, D.M., Davis, R.B., Ettner, S.L., Appel, S., Wilkey, S., Van Rompay, M., *et al.* (1998) Trends in alternative medicine use in the United States, 1990–1997: Results of a follow-up national survey. *Journal of the American Medical Association* 280 (18), 1569–1575.

Kwong, E.Y-L. and Yiu, E.M-L. (2010) A preliminary study of the effect of acupuncture on emotional stress in female dysphonic speakers. *Journal of Voice* 24 (6), 719–723.

Ma, E.P-M. and Yiu, E.M-L. (2001) Voice activity and participation profile: Assessing the impact of voice disorders on daily activities. *Journal of Speech, Language, and Hearing Research* 44 (3), 511–524.

Ma, E. and Yiu, E. (2005) Suitability of acoustic perturbation measures in analyzing periodic and nearly periodic voice signals. *Folia Phoniatrica et Logopaedica* 57 (1), 38–47.

Ma, E., Robertson, J., Radford, C., Vagne, S., El-Halabi, R. and Yiu, E. (2007) Reliability of speaking and maximum voice range measures in screening for dysphonia. *Journal of Voice* 21 (4), 397–406.

MacKenzie, K., Millar, A., Wilson, J.A., Sellars, C. and Deary, I.J. (2001) Is voice therapy an effective treatment for dysphonia? A randomised controlled trial. *British Medical Journal* 323 (7314), 658–661.

Mann, F. (1983) *Scientific Aspects of Acupuncture*. London: William Heinemann Medical.

Mann, F. (1992) *Acupuncture: Cure of Many Diseases* (2nd edn). Oxford: Butterworth-Heinemann.

Naeser, M.A., Alexander, M.P., Stiassny-Eder, D., Galler, V., Hobbs, J., Bachman, D., *et al.* (1995) Laser acupuncture in the treatment of paralysis in stroke patients – a CT scan lesion site study. *American Journal of Acupuncture* 23 (1), 13–28.

Radmayr, C., Schlager, A., Studen, M. and Bartsch, G. (2001) Prospective randomized trial using laser acupuncture versus desmopressin in the treatment of nocturnal enuresis. *European Urology* 40, 201–205.

Ramig, L.O. and Verdolini, K. (1998) Treatment efficacy: Voice disorders. *Journal of Speech, Language, and Hearing Research* 41, S101–S116.

Ricarte, A., Gasparini, G. and Behlau, M. (2006) Validação do Protocolo Perfil de Participação e Atividades Vocais (PPAV) no Brasil. *Anais do XIV Congresso Brasileiro de Fonoaudiologia.*

Rubin, J.S. and Yanagisawa, E. (2003) Benign vocal fold pathology through the eyes of the laryngologist. In J.S. Rubin, R.T. Sataloff and G.S. Korovin (eds) *Diagnosis and Treatment of Voice Disorders* (2nd edn). New York: Thomson Learning.

Stokes, S.F. and Yiu, E. (1997) Speech therapy and general practice in Hong Kong. *Hong Kong Practitioner* 19 (7), 374–379.

Sukanen, O., Sihvo, M., Rorarius, E., Lehtihalmes, M., Autio, V. and Kleemola, L. (2007) Voice Activity and Participation Profile (VAPP) in assessing the effects of voice disorders on patients' quality of life: Validity and reliability of the Finnish version of VAPP. *Logopedics Phoniatrics Vocology* 32, 3–8.

WHO (2002) *WHO Traditional Medicine Strategy 2002–2005*. Geneva: World Health Organization.

Woo, P., Casper, J., Colton, R. and Brewer, D. (1994) Diagnosis and treatment of persistence dysphonia after laryngeal surgery: A retrospective analysis of 62 patients. *Laryngoscope* 104, 1084–1091.

Wozniak, P., Stachowiak, G., Pieta-Dolinska, A. and Oszukowski, P. (2003) Laser acupuncture and low-calorie diet during visceral obesity therapy after menopause. *Acta Obstetricia et Gynecologica Scandinavica* 82, 69–73.

Yang, S. (2000) Clinical observations on 109 cases of vocal nodules treated with acupuncture and Chinese drugs. *Journal of Traditional Medicine* 20 (3), 202–205.

Yao, W. (2000) Prof. Shen Canruo's experience in acupuncture treatment of throat diseases with Yan Si Xue. *Journal of Traditional Medicine* 20 (2), 122–125.

Yiu, E.M-L., Yuen, Y.M., Whitehill, T. and Winkworth, A. (2004) Reliability and applicability of aerodynamic measures in dysphonia assessment. *Clinical Linguistics and Phonetics* 18 (6–8), 463–478.

Yiu, E.M-L., Verdolini, K. and Chow, L.P-Y. (2005) Electromyographic study of motor learning for a voice production task. *Journal of Speech, Language, and Hearing Research* 48, 1254–1268.

Yiu, E.M-L., Xu, J.J., Murry, T., Wei, W., Yu, M., Ma, E., Huang, W. and Kwong E. (2006) A randomized treatment–placebo study of the effectiveness of acupuncture for benign vocal pathologies. *Journal of Voice* 20, 144–156.

Yiu, E.M-L., Chan, K.M.K. and Mok, R.S-M. (2007) Reliability and confidence in using a paired comparison paradigm in perceptual voice quality evaluation. *Clinical Linguistics and Phonetics* 21 (2), 129–145.

Yiu, E.M-L., Kong, J-P., Fong, R. and Chan, K.M-K. (2010) A preliminary study of a quantitative analysis method for high-speed laryngoscopic images. *International Journal of Speech-Language Pathology* 12 (6), 520–528.

Yiu, E.M-L., Kwong, E., Chan, K.M-K., Verdolini-Abbot, K., Lin, Z., Tse, W., *et al.* (in progress) A double-blind randomized control trial of acupuncture treatment for benign phonotraumatic vocal fold pathologies.

# 14 Application of Motor Learning Principles in Voice Motor Learning

## Estella P-M. Ma and Edwin M-L. Yiu

## General Background

Hyperfunctional or phonotraumatic voice disorders are among the most common types of voice disorder seen at voice clinics in Hong Kong (Yiu & Ho, 1991) and worldwide (Andrews, 1996; Redenbaugh & Reich, 1989). Hyperfunctional voice disorder is characterized by an excessive muscle tension in the perilaryngeal area during phonation. Conservative behavioral therapy is generally considered as the first treatment option for hyperfunctional voice disorders. Behavioral voice therapy usually includes vocal hygiene education and vocal facilitative techniques to improve vocal efficiency. Training using vocal facilitative techniques aims at reducing muscle tension in the perilaryngeal area for more effective phonation (Greene & Mathieson, 1989; Lo, 2000).

The effectiveness of behavioral voice therapy has been demonstrated in many studies (see reviews by Pannbacker, 1998; Ramig & Verdolini, 1998). However, very little is known about the 'learning' process of the therapeutic techniques. Data from the general, non-speech motor learning literature suggest that learning processes can be facilitated (or hindered) by manipulating different learning variables during training. Therefore, practitioners involved in voice therapy are keen to find out specifically how the learning of voice motor skills can be facilitated. Since the beginning of 2000, the Voice Research Laboratory at the University of Hong Kong has developed a series of research programs on voice motor learning which examine the application of general motor learning principles in voice motor learning. The research program aims to develop a voice training protocol which explicates more effective training methods and practice strategies for the learning and the acquisition of voice motor tasks. The following sections will discuss three voice motor learning variables carried out at the Voice Research Laboratory at the University of Hong Kong: task instructions, structure of practice and a feedback paradigm.

In order to understand voice motor learning, an operational definition of motor learning is needed. Motor learning is defined as a set of processes that can lead to relatively permanent changes in motor performance, as the result of practice or experience (Schmidt & Lee, 1999). Therefore, learning should be assessed using long-term retention tests rather than performance during training.

## Task instructions

It is generally assumed that explicit biomechanical instructions are necessary to learn how to produce the desirable vocal qualities in voice therapy. For example, a clinician may instruct the client to produce a smooth phonation onset using the yawn-sigh technique, with the instruction: 'Open your mouth wide, pull the tongue back and inhale as deeply as possible. While breathing out, say the prolonged/ha/ with the mouth widely opened.' From a theoretical perspective, providing explicit biomechanical information about the motor skill at the beginning of practice helps the learner to establish a reference of correctness (Swinnen, 1996). With this biomechanical information, it is assumed that learners would be able to detect their errors while performing the task, and evaluate their own performance from time to time. However, the benefits of providing explicit instructions on physical principles in motor learning have been questioned by the implicit motor learning literature (Hardy et al., 1996; Hodges & Lee, 1999; Masters, 1992; Wulf & Weigelt, 1997). Evidence from the literature suggests that providing learners with explicit instructions on how to perform a motor task may not always be effective. In fact, the provision of explicit instructions and strategies to learn the skill can degrade learning when compared to other participants who are not informed about the strategies.

A number of researchers have suggested that the manipulation of task instructions can result in different modes of learning (Berry, 1993; Berry & Broadbent, 1988; Berry & Dienes, 1993; Hodges & Lee, 1999; Jacoby et al., 1993). When explicit instructions and knowledge on *what and how* to perform the task are given, learners are directed to use the strategies instructed to acquire the skill in the task. They may therefore limit their exploration of different possible strategies to achieve the task. This learning mode has been referred as explicit learning (Berry, 1993; Berry & Broadbent, 1988). On the other hand, by simply mentioning to the learner *'what'* to achieve in the task (that is, the target) without telling the learner *'how'* to perform the task, learners may explore different strategies to acquire the skill. They may discover several possible strategies and use the optimal one(s) to meet the target. This learning mode has been referred to as discovery learning (Hodges & Lee, 1999; Vereijken & Whiting, 1990).

The effects of the provision of explicit task instructions have been demonstrated on gross motor skill learning (Hodges & Lee, 1999; Wulf & Weigelt, 1997). The performances of learners who were given explicit instructions were compared with those who were not given any instructions. These studies showed that providing learners explicitly with specific biomechanical instructions on how to perform the task tends to degrade learning. Wulf and Weigelt (1997) investigated how learners learnt skiing-like movements on a ski simulator. Participants stood on a platform that could be moved from side to side. Their goal in the task was to make the fastest sideways movements of the platform with the greatest amplitude. One group of learners were explicitly told about the underlying rules and principles governing their performance. They were instructed about the optimal timing to exert force on the platform in order to perform the task effectively. Another group of learners, who were given a discovery learning condition, were simply asked to perform the task and they were not given any specific strategies. The participants under the discovery learning mode were found to perform better throughout the training period when compared to the participants under the explicit learning condition. The participants who learned through the discovery learning condition also achieved better performance in the transfer test in which learners were required to perform the same skiing task under a stressful situation (participants were told that their performance would be evaluated by a skiing expert).

Similar findings have been reported by Hodges and Lee (1999). In their study, participants were required to learn a complex dual limb coordination task which involved coordinating their hands 90 degrees out of phase in making a circle pattern displayed on a computer monitor. One group of participants was provided with the underlying physical principles to perform the coordination task efficiently. Another group was just asked to perform the task without the provision of any specific instructions. Results showed that the participants who were not given any instructions performed better during training and in the retention test.

The Voice Research Laboratory at the University of Hong Kong has conducted a study to investigate whether the provision of explicit and detailed instructions can affect voice motor learning (Ma & Cheung, 2009). In this study, task instructions were given on the underlying biomechanical knowledge and strategies needed to achieve relaxed phonation. Twenty-six vocally healthy participants were randomly assigned to two practice groups: a group with explicit instructions and a group with minimal instruction. The two groups underwent identical training except in the amount and nature of instructions. In the minimal instruction group, the participants were only told about the target of the task (that is, relaxed phonation). However, they were not given any additional instructions regarding how to achieve relaxed phonation. Electromyographic (EMG) waveform regarding the degree of neck muscle tension was provided. In the explicit instruction group, detailed instructions on how to achieve a relaxed phonation using chant-talk and the open mouth approach (Ma, 2008) were given.

Throughout the training, participants in the explicit instruction group were reminded to use the vocal facilitative technique to produce relaxed voicing in every eight sentences (that is, the first, eighth and 16th sentence of each training block). Participants in the minimal instruction group were simply reminded about the target, that is, to minimize the EMG waveform amplitudes. Both groups received terminal visual feedback from the EMG system in the form of a static EMG display after reading aloud every two sentences (see Cheung, 2004; Yiu *et al.*, 2005). Throughout the training, the vocal intensity was monitored and maintained by a sound level meter.

The results revealed different learning patterns across time between the two groups of learners (Figure 14.1). For the explicit instruction group, their EMG amplitudes reduced sharply from the baseline to the acquisition phase but in the retention phases the amplitudes regressed to the baseline level. The minimal instruction group demonstrated a progressive decrease in EMG amplitudes across baseline, acquisition and retention test phases. These results suggested that participants in the explicit instruction group were not able to maintain their performance during training in the retention phases. Participants in the minimal instruction group were able to maintain their performance during training in the retention phases, and learning had occurred in this group of participants.

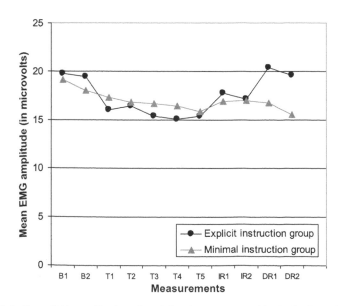

**Figure 14.1** Mean EMG amplitudes of training list across 11 blocks in four time phases
Notes: B, baseline; T, training; IR, immediate retention; DR, delayed retention.

The different learning patterns of the two groups could possibly be due to the use of different learning strategies to achieve relaxed voicing. During the acquisition phase, the explicit instruction group might have concentrated on the technique as instructed to reduce excessive laryngeal muscle tension. Their EMG amplitudes reduced sharply from the baseline to the acquisition phase with this effective strategy. On the contrary, the minimal instruction group were not directed towards any specific technique to produce relaxed phonation. They might have been more proactive in exploring the task dynamics and discovering an optimal way to perform the task effectively. While they were exploring how to produce relaxed phonation, their EMG amplitudes did not reduce as quickly as the explicit instruction group did during the acquisition phase. At the retention phases, the explicit instruction group were not able to maintain relaxed voicing. Their EMG amplitudes regressed to the baseline levels. It is possible that the explicit instruction group had not internalized the relaxed phonation skills and hence were not able to maintain relaxed voicing. On the other hand, participants in the minimal instruction group might have gathered important information about the sensory processes of relaxed phonation through their exploration process. Such information facilitated them in maintaining relaxed voicing skills in the retention tests.

## Structure of practice

Another learning variable that is central to any motor therapy is the structure of practice. Evidence in the learning literature has shown that motor learning is enhanced by the use of variable practice items, as opposed to using a constant set of stimuli or practicing on a few repeating stimuli (that is, non-variable practice) (McCracken & Stelmach, 1977). It is believed that variable practice conditions produce higher contextual interference and hence promote learning. Shea and Morgan (1979) showed that adults learned better in a motor task when the practice items were presented in a randomized rather than a constant fashion. Similar findings were reported by Wulf and Schmidt (1997). Wulf (1991) examined learning a novel motor task in children under different practice paradigms. Her results revealed that children who received variable practice demonstrated the best performance during retention, rather than children who received less variable practice. Recently, Porter and Magill (2010) studied the use of a mixed practice schedule with a systematic increase in the level of contextual interference (blocked practice followed by random practice) in the learning of golf-putting. They found that participants under this mixed practice schedule performed better learning than those who received either a random or a blocked practice schedule. In speech motor learning, Knock and colleagues (2000) found that random practice conditions facilitated a better re-learning of speech production skills than those who received blocked practice conditions, in adults with acquired apraxia of speech. The benefits of using variable practice over constant practice are also demonstrated in a study by Adams and Page (2000), which compared the learning benefits of practicing under constant or variable conditions in healthy adults on a speech motor task. Another study in speech motor learning also demonstrated better learning in practice conditions which required more cognitive loading on the participant (Wong et al., submitted). In their study, participants were asked to learn how to produce a Cantonese phrase at different speech rates. Four practice conditions were used: blocked, random and two mixed practice conditions (blocked-then-variable and variable-then-blocked). The results revealed that the performances of participants in the mixed practice conditions were more resistant (hence, better learning) at transfer tests involving secondary task.

A voice motor learning study was carried out at the Voice Research Laboratory to evaluate the effects of practice variability (Wong et al., 2011). Twenty-four voice-disordered individuals were randomly assigned to a constant practice group, blocked practice group and random practice group. All participants were asked to learn reading aloud sentence stimuli using a relaxed voice. Surface EMG was used to provide augmented visual feedback during training. Participants in the constant practice group were asked to practice reading aloud sentence stimuli with four Cantonese characters. Participants in the blocked practice group were asked to read aloud sentence stimuli with increasing sentence length, starting from sets of two characters up to five characters. Participants in the random practice group were asked to practice reading sentence stimuli of variable length presented in a random fashion. Results did not reveal any significant difference in the reduction of EMG values among the three practice groups. The results were interpreted as attributable to the high complexity and difficulty of the phonation task for dysphonic participants.

## Feedback paradigm

Feedback is another learning variable that has gained much attention in the learning literature. Feedback can be manipulated in terms of the relative frequency (100%, 50%, 0%; see Steinhauer & Grayhack, 2000) and timing (concurrent versus terminal; see Yiu et al., 2005). One feedback paradigm that has gained increasing interest is the self-controlled feedback paradigm, and this will be discussed in the following sections.

The traditional voice training model takes a clinician-directed approach. Under this approach, the clinician is the key person to determine practice variables during training, namely the schedule of practice and feedback. The learners have minimal control in the planning process of the training and their role is relatively passive. Interestingly, studies in the general motor learning literature have demonstrated that increasing learners' control over practice conditions has a positive influence on the learning of motor skills.

It is suggested that learners who have more control in manipulating practice variables take a more active role in the learning process itself. Such a self-controlled learning paradigm promotes more cognitive processing and hence better learning. Under this self-controlled learning paradigm, the learner has some control over different practice parameters such as the schedule of provision of feedback.

The role and benefits of self-control on motor skills learning have been examined and demonstrated by Janelle and colleagues using a ball-tossing task (Janelle et al., 1995, 1997). Wulf and Toole (1999) demonstrated the benefits of self-control in the use of physical assistance devices. Similar encouraging findings were reported by Chiviacowsky and Wulf (2002). They compared the self-controlled feedback paradigm with external, clinician-controlled feedback paradigms in a sequential timing task. Their findings revealed that learners who could decide when they wanted to receive feedback about their performance performed significantly better in the retention test, and hence gained better learning, than their yoked counterparts. In summary, the reports of the benefits of using a self-controlled learning paradigm showed very satisfactory results in limb motor learning.

The Voice Research Laboratory conducted a study to examine the effects of the self-controlled feedback paradigm on voice motor learning (Ma et al., submitted). Twenty-four vocally healthy individuals participated to learn how to produce 'relaxed phonation'. Half of them were assigned to a self-controlled feedback group, and the other half of them were assigned to a yoked (control) group. Participants in the self-controlled feedback group were told that they would receive visual feedback on their performance only when they requested it. Participants in the yoked group had no such option. The feedback presentation schedule of each yoked participant was based on that of the corresponding matched participant in the self-controlled group.

Results revealed that both the self-controlled and yoked groups improved significantly across time. For both groups of participants, motor learning was evidenced by a significant decrease in EMG levels in the delayed retention test. It was apparent that the type of feedback paradigm did not seem to have any significant effects on the learning of the voice task. One possible reason for the lack of group difference might have been due to the high percentage of feedback requested by the self-controlled participants. On average, participants in the self-controlled group requested feedback for over two-thirds of all training trials. It is possible that, during training, participants in the self-controlled group actively set out a hypothesis based on their vocal performance and the feedback they received. Such hypothesis testing could have caused the learners to correct their own performance more consciously and therefore hampered their learning (see Masters & Maxwell, 2004, for review). On the other hand, the yoked group did not know when feedback would be provided. The possibility of setting out and evaluating a hypothesis was minimized in the yoked group.

## Conclusion and Future Research Agenda

In conclusion, our program of research on voice motor learning suggests that general motor learning principles may not always be applicable to the learning of vocal skills. Further voice motor learning research should be carried out with different populations (e.g. children versus adults). Children are different from adults in their cognitive ability and their amount of motor experience with different motor skills. Therefore, findings from adult speakers may not necessarily be applicable to children. In summary, this line of research could help to refine the procedural aspects of voice therapy, by informing voice clinicians about the instructional settings that facilitate the learning of motor skills.

## Acknowledgements

Part of this chapter was adapted from the publications arising from research supported in part by two research grants awarded by the Hong Kong Research Grant Council General Research Fund (HKU 7451/06H and HKU 7486/08H).

## References

Adams, S.G. and Page, A.D. (2000) Effects of selected practice and feedback variables on speech motor learning. *Journal of Medical Speech-Language Pathology* 8, 215–220.

Andrews, M.L. (1996) Treatment of vocal hyperfunction in adolescents. *Language, Speech, and Hearing Services in Schools* 27, 251–256.

Berry, D. (1993) The control of complex systems. In D.C. Berry & Z. Dienes (eds) *Implicit Learning: Theoretical and Empirical Issues*. Hove: Lawrence Erlbaum Associates.

Berry, D. and Broadbent, D. (1988) Interactive tasks and the implicit-explicit distinction. *British Journal of Psychology* 79, 251–272.

Berry, D. and Dienes, Z. (1993) Towards a working characterization of implicit learning. In D.C. Berry and Z. Dienes (eds) *Implicit Learning: Theoretical and Empirical Issues*. Hove: Lawrence Erlbaum Associates.

Cheung, C.P.S. (2004) The effect of continuous versus fading feedback on laryngeal muscle relaxation learning. Unpublished BSc dissertation, University of Hong Kong.

Chiviacowsky, S. and Wulf, G. (2002) Self-controlled feedback: Does it enhance learning because performers get feedback when they need it? *Research Quarterly for Exercise and Sport* 73, 408–415.

Greene, M.C.L. and Mathieson, L. (1989) *The Voice and its Disorders* (5th edn). London: Whurr Publishers.

Hardy, L., Mullen, R. and Jones, G. (1996) Knowledge and conscious control of motor actions under stress. *British Journal of Psychology* 87, 621–636.

Hodges, N.J. and Lee, T.D. (1999) The role of augmented information prior to learning a bimanual visual-motor coordination task: Do instructions of the movement pattern facilitate learning relative to discovery learning? *British Journal of Psychology* 90, 389–403.

Jacoby, L.L., Ste-Marie, D. and Toth, J.P. (1993) Redefining automaticity: Unconscious influences, awareness, and control. In A. Baddeley and L. Weiskrantz (eds) *Attention: Selection, Awareness, and Control*. Oxford: Oxford University Press.

Janelle, C.M., Kim, J. and Singer, R.N. (1995) Subject-controlled performance feedback and learning of a closed motor skill. *Perceptual and Motor Skills* 81, 627–634.

Janelle, C.M., Barba, D.A., Frehlich, S.G., Tennant, L.K. and Cauraugh, J.H. (1997) Maximizing performance feedback effectiveness through videotape replay and a self-controlled environment. *Research Quarterly of Exercise and Sport* 68, 269–279.

Knock, T.R., Ballard, K.J. and Schmidt, R.A. (2000) Influence of order of stimulus presentation on speech motor learning: A principled approach to treatment for apraxia of speech. *Aphasiology* 14 (5–6), 653–668.

Lo, C.O-Y. (2000) Differences in management strategies for hyperfunctional voice disorders between speech therapists and student speech therapists. Unpublished BSc dissertation, University of Hong Kong.

Ma, E. (2008) Chewing technique: Speak with an 'open mouth'. In A. Behrman and J. Haskell (eds) *Exercises for Voice Therapy* (pp. 85–86). San Diego: Plural Publishing.

Ma, E. and Cheung, O. (2009) The effects of task instructions on the learning of relaxed phonation. Paper presented at *The Voice Foundation's 38th Annual Symposium*, Philadelphia.

Ma, E.P-M., Yiu, G.K-Y. and Yiu, E.M-L. (submitted) Effects of self-controlled learning on the learning of 'relaxed phonation' task. *Journal of Voice*.

Masters, R.S.W. (1992) Knowledge, knerves and know-how. *British Journal of Psychology* 83, 343–358.

Masters, R.S.W. and Maxwell, J.P. (2004) Implicit motor learning, reinvestment and movement disruption: What you don't know won't hurt you? In A.M. Williams and N.J. Hodges (eds) *Skill Acquisition in Sport: Research, Theory and Practice*. London: Routledge.

McCracken, H.D. and Stelmach, G.E. (1977) A test of schema theory of discrete motor learning. *Journal of Motor Behaviour* 9, 193–201.

Pannbacker, M. (1998) Voice treatment techniques: A review and recommendations for outcome studies. *American Journal of Speech-Language Pathology* 7 (3), 49–64.

Porter, J.M. and Magill, R.A. (2010) Systematically increasing contextual interference is beneficial for learning sport skills. *Journal of Sports Sciences* 28, 1277–1285.

Ramig, L.O. and Verdolini, K. (1998) Treatment efficacy: Voice disorders. *Journal of Speech, Language, and Hearing Research* 41, S101–S116.

Redenbaugh, M.A. and Reich, A.R. (1989) Surface EMG and related measures in normal and vocally hyperfunctional speakers. *Journal of Speech and Hearing Disorders* 54, 68–73.

Schmidt, R.A. and Lee, T.D. (1999) *Motor Control and Learning: A Behavioural Emphasis* (3rd edn). Champaign: Human Kinetics.

Shea, J.B. and Morgan, R.L. (1979) Contextual interference effects on the acquisition, retention, and transfer of a motor skill. *Journal of Experimental Psychology: Human Learning and Memory* 5, 179–187.

Steinhauer, K. and Grayhack, J.P. (2000) The role of knowledge of results in performance and learning of a voice motor task. *Journal of Voice* 14 (2), 137–145.

Swinnen, S.P. (1996) Information feedback for motor skill learning: A review. In H.N. Zelaznik (ed.) *Advances in Motor Learning and Control*. Champaign: Human Kinetics.

Vereijken, B. and Whiting, H.T.A. (1990) In defence of discovery learning. *Canadian Journal of Sport Sciences* 15, 99–106.

Wong, A.Y-H., Ma, E.P-M. and Yiu, E.M-L. (2011) Effects of practice variability on learning of relaxed phonation in vocally hyperfunctional speakers. *Journal of Voice* 25, 103–113.

Wong, A.W-K., Whitehill, T.L., Ma, E.P-M. and Masters, R. (submitted) Effects of practice schedules on speech motor learning. *International Journal of Speech-Language Pathology*.

Wulf, G. (1991) The effect of type of practice on motor learning in children. *Applied Cognitive Psychology* 5, 123–134.

Wulf, G. and Schmidt, R.A. (1997) Variability of practice and implicit motor learning. *Journal of Experimental Psychology: Learning, Memory, and Cognition* 23 (4), 987–1006.

Wulf, G. and Toole, T. (1999) Physical assistance devices in complex motor skill learning: Benefits of a self-controlled practice schedule. *Research Quarterly for Exercise and Sport* 70, 265–272.

Wulf, G. and Weigelt, C. (1997) Instructions about physical principles in learning a complex motor skill: To tell or not to tell …. *Research Quarterly for Exercise and Sport* 68 (4), 362–367.

Yiu, E.M-L. and Ho, P.S-P. (1991) Voice problems in Hong Kong: A preliminary report. *Australian Journal of Human Communication Disorders* 19, 45–58.

Yiu, E.M-L., Verdolini, K. and Chow, L.P-Y. (2005) Electromyographic study of motor learning for a voice production task. *Journal of Speech, Language and Hearing Research* 48, 1254–1268.

# 15 Contemporary Voice Research: A China Perspective

Jiangping Kong and Gaowu Wang

## Current Voice Research in China

The study of speech and voice has a long history in China. As early as the Song Dynasty, a polymath scholar named Shen Kuo (1031–1095) documented the application of an artificial larynx in his famous book entitled 'Mengxi Bi Tan' (written in the Mengxi Garden):

> Devices made by people from materials, such as bamboo, wood, ivory and bone, were called sound generators. A sound generator, which could be put into the throat and produce speech sound by whistling, was called a voice generator. A dumb person, who suffered from injustice, could not argue in court for himself. The judge let people put a voice generator in his throat, and asked him to speak. The speech articulated like puppet talk, but could roughly make sense. His injustice was finally redressed.

This script vividly depicted the case of an artificial larynx and its forensic application in ancient China. With the development of science and technology, the study of speech and voice has advanced across a number of disciplines, such as linguistics, medicine and speech engineering. In China, the linguists and phoneticians have a strong interest in voice science research. This chapter will introduce current voice research in China from the linguists' perspective in the areas of: (1) language phonation types in China; (2) methods for studying voice; and (3) the studies of phonation types in different Chinese languages.

## Language Phonation Types in China

There are more than 80 languages used in China. Many of them use multiple phonation types to convey meaning. These Chinese languages include

Mongolian, Tibetan, Uigur, Bai, Yi, Korean, Hani, Western Yugur, Zhuang, Miao (Hmong), Wa (Va), Sui, Zaiwa (Atsi) and Jingpho. Although these phonation phenomena have been noticed by linguists for a long time, they have not been studied specifically or scientifically, possibly due to the lack of relevant technologies. The phonemic meanings conveyed by these phonation types have been described phonetically and studied from the perspective of historical comparative linguistics. These studies are listed in Table 15.1.

# Methods for Studying Voicing (Phonation Types)

Speech signal, electroglottography (EGG) and high-speed digital imaging (HSDI) have been used in China to study the voicing characteristics of the different Chinese language phonation types. Speech signal analyses include harmonic analysis, inverse filtering, spectrum descent or tilt, multidimensional voice processing and voice range profile.

## Harmonic analysis

Harmonic analysis estimates the phonation types according to the energy of the first harmonic (H1), the second harmonic (H2) and their ratio (H2/H1). In the 1970s, phoneticians from North America studied the phonation types in a number of languages using harmonic analysis (Kirk et al., 1984; Kong, 2001b; Ladefoged, 1973, 1988; Ladefoged et al., 1987, 1988; Laver, 1980; Maddieson & Ladefoged, 1985; Thongkum, 1988; Traill & Jackson, 1988). One of the limitations of this method is that the resonant formants in the speech spectrum would inadvertently alter the energy of each harmonic. The employment of the vowel /a/ for harmonic study minimizes the influences on the harmonics in the low-frequency region as the first formant of /a/ has a relatively high frequency.

## Inverse filtering

In inverse filtering, the speech signal is filtered by a processor which has the inverse resonant property of the original source. In modern signal processing, the linear prediction coefficient (LPC) can be used to estimate the resonant properties effectively (Alku, 1992; Fant & Gauffin, 1994; Lindestad et al., 2001).

## Spectrum descent/tilt

Normally, the spectrum of human voice signal reduces by 12 dB per octave. This is called spectrum descent/tilt. This tilt is affected by the gender of the speaker, the language, as well as the phonation type. Spectrum tilt analysis generally includes: (1) obtaining the sound source signal by inverse filtering; (2) calculating the power spectrum frame-by-frame and detecting

**Table 15.1** Phonetic and linguistic studies of ethnic languages in China

| Family | Branch | Group | Language | Spoken population | Language phonation | Linguistic study |
|---|---|---|---|---|---|---|
| Sino-Tibetan | Tibeto-Burman | Yi | Hani | 1,500,000 | 10 tense/lax vowels | Li and Wang (1986) |
| | | | Nu | 23,000 | 8 tense/2 creaky vowels | Sun and Liu (1986) |
| | | | Bai | 820,000 | Tense/lax tones | Xu and Zhao (1984) |
| | | | Lisu | 500,000 | Tense/lax tones | Xu et al. (1986) |
| | | | Lahu | 300,000 | Tense vowels | Chang (1986) |
| | | Jingpo | Jingpho | 90,000 | 5 tense & 5 lax vowels | Liu (1984) |
| | | Burmish | Zaiwa | 90,000 | 5 tense & 5 lax vowels | Xu and Xu (1984) |
| | Miao-Yao | Miao | Miao | 6,000,000 | Voiced aspirated initials | Wang (1985) |
| | Austro-Asiatic | Palaung-Wa | Wa | 270,000 | 9 tense & 9 lax vowels | Zhou and Yan (1984) |
| Altaic | Mongolic | Mongolic | Mongolian | 3,400,000 | 7 tense & 12 lax vowels | Dao (1983) |
| | Turkic | Eastern Turkic | Western Yugur | 1,000,000 | Fricative vowels | Chen and Lei (1984) |
| | | | Korean | 1,700,000 | Tense/lax consonants | Xuan et al. (1985) |

Notes: FU2, follow-up 2; FU3, follow-up 3.

the local maximum power in each frame; (3) performing apolynomial fit on each local maximum power; and (4) calculating the spectrum tilt, that is, how much the fitting curve decreases (in dB) per octave.

## Multidimensional voice analysis

Multidimensional voice processing is a method used to evaluate voice quality using a group of acoustic measurements. These may include fundamental frequency (F0), standard deviation of F0 (STD), jitter and shimmer. An example of such a method is the Kay–Pentax Multi-Dimensional Voice Program. It is generally believed that a single measurement alone is not enough to describe the voice quality adequately. Using a multitude of measurements is presumably a better way to assess a more comprehensive voice quality profile. We found that multidimensional analysis is a useful tool to study phonation types (Hall & Yairi, 1992; Horii, 1985; Kong, 2001b; Kong et al., 1997; Shen & Kong, 1998).

## Electroglottographic analysis

EGG is a non-invasive measurement which provides information on the degree of contact between the two vibrating vocal folds during voice production (Caodao & Kong, 1999; Childers et al., 1990; Dickson et al., 1994; Holmberg et al., 1995; Kong, 1999, 2001a; Orlikoff, 1991; Rothenberg & Mahshie, 1988; Shen & Kong, 1999).

The measurements extracted from the EGG signals can be used to study the relationships among glottal variations (opening/closing, vibration of vocal folds and voice source). This is useful for studying language phonation types. Three measurements are particularly useful in EGG analysis: (1) fundamental frequency, (2) open quotient (OQ) and (3) speed quotient (SQ). F0 is the reciprocal of glottal period, OQ is the ratio of open phase over the whole glottal period, and SQ is the ratio of opening phase over the closing phase. These measurements can also be extracted from the speech signal.

These three measurements can be used to describe and define phonation types. In phonetics, the 'acoustic diagram of vowels' is used to describe the position and property of vowels. In voice, we propose an 'acoustic diagram of voice' (see Figure 15.1) to describe the properties of phonation types (Kong, 2001b). The concept of the acoustic diagram of voice has been used to study the Sutra Chanting of Tibetan Buddhism (Yoshinaga & Kong, 2011). In Figure 15.1, the black circles denote the voice samples in Sutra chanting, and the gray circles denote the voice samples in modal voices. It can be seen that the Sutra chanting of Tibetan Buddhism is significantly different from modal voices with respect to the three voice measurements (F0, OQ and SQ).

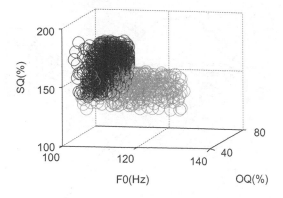

**Figure 15.1** Acoustic diagram of voice
Notes: F0, fundamental frequency; SQ, speed quotient; OQ, open quotient.

## Imaging of the dynamic glottis

Imaging techniques have also been used in the study of speech and voice production. An earlier example which prominently marked the focus of modern scientific phonetics is the use of X-ray imaging in experimental phonetics to explore the relationship between tongue position and speech articulation. The invention of high-speed imaging in the 1980s has allowed the direct observation and analysis of the glottal vibration (Kiritani *et al.*, 1993).

Figure 15.2 illustrates the acquisition of signals through three channels: high-speed images, speech signal and EGG signal. The sample rate of high-speed imaging used by Kiritani *et al.* (1993) was 4501 frames per second (fps), in $256 \times 256$ pixels and 8-bit grayscale. With the advance in computer speed and memory capacity, contemporary high-speed systems could have a frame rate as high as 9000 fps and images captured in color.

Since high-speed images contain a huge amount (2000–9000 fps) of information, different methods have been reported to process the captured images. We will outline the processing method described by Kong and Yiu (2011). Figure 15.3 outlines the procedure of image processing. The images are first pre-processed to align the axis of the image, to reduce image background noise and to compensate for any motion caused by the camera. This will provide appropriate images of the glottis for quantitative analysis. A rectangular window is added manually to the pre-processed images to cover the glottis. Then the images are adjusted for brightness and contrast, and finally binarized, manually or automatically.

A number of glottal measurements can be extracted from these high-speed images (Kong, 2007; Kong & Yiu, 2011). These include, for example, the glottal total area, left/right glottal area (GA), glottal total width, maximum of GA, OQ and SQ.

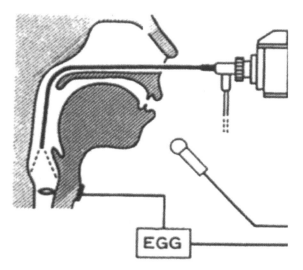

**Figure 15.2** Acquisition of high-speed image, acoustic and electroglottal signals (Kiritani *et al.*, 1993)

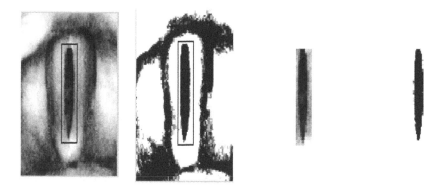

**Figure 15.3** An illustration of image processing (Kong, 2007)

# Voice Characteristics of Phonation Types in Chinese Languages

Scientists in China have undertaken a number of studies on the voice characteristics of different phonation types in different Chinese languages.

## Tense/lax phonation in the Hani language

In the Dazhai dialect of the Hani Language in Luchun County, there are 31 initials, 26 finals and four lexical tones, and tense/lax phonations (Kong,

1996). It was generally agreed among the Chinese linguists that, during the production of tense vowels, the laryngeal muscles contract, with short and fast airflow, and resonating vowels; during the production of lax vowels, the laryngeal muscles are slacked, with smooth airflow and less resonating vowels (Li & Wang, 1986). Ladefoged (Ladefoged et al., 1988; Maddieson & Ladefoged, 1985) contended that the ratio of aspiration to pressure is higher during the production of lax vowels.

Kong (1996) found that the tense vowels were produced in a creaky voice but lax vowels were produced in modal voice, and the first formant (F1) in the tense vowels was higher than that in the lax vowels. There were no significant differences between the tone pitch in lax and tense vowels and the syllable length of a lax vowel was longer than that of tense vowel.

## Voiced aspiration in the Miao language

The Shimenkan dialect of the Miao language has 56 initials, 21 finals and eight lexical tones (Wang, 1985). In addition, voiced aspiration in the Miao language is also phonemic in nature, that is, it signifies meaning. Voice aspiration has been treated as fricative vowels or a low lexical tone by some experts.

From his study of voice aspiration, Kong (2001b) found that voiced aspiration was a breathy voice production and the pitch of the tones in voiced aspiration was lower than that of the unvoiced aspiration. In addition, the difference between harmonic 1 and harmonic 2 (H1–H2) on the onsets of vowels in syllables was higher when aspirated.

## Tense/lax voices in the Liangshan Yi language

The Liangshan dialect of the Yi language has 43 initials, 10 finals, four tones and tense/lax vowels. It has been reported that the phonation type of lax vowels is modal but that of tense vowels is creaky (Maddieson & Hess, 1986; Maddieson & Ladefoged, 1985). Kong (2001b) studied the relationship between the phonation type and the shape of the vocal tract. He found that lax vowels were produced by a higher tongue position when compared with their tense counterparts; the posterior part of the vocal tract compressed relatively more than the anterior part in the production of tense vowels. Thus, the differences between lax and tense vowel production in the Liangshan dialect can be detected by looking at the differing tension of the vocal folds, the configuration of the pharyngeal cavity and the position of the tongue. Tense vowel phonation has a creaky voice, tensed vocal folds and muscles, and forward positioning of the tongue which results in a relatively large pharyngeal space.

## Tense/lax voices in the Axi Yi language

The Axi dialect of Yi language has 29 initials, 16 finals, three tones, and tense/lax vowel phonation types (Wu, 1981). The distinctive features of tense/lax voices in the Axi dialect are similar to those described above (Kong, 2001b).

## Phonation types in the Zaiwa language

The Zaiwa language has 28 initials, 86 finals and three tones. There are five tense and five lax vowels in the Zaiwa language, which are treated as different phonation types from the aspects of acoustics and physiology. Kong (2001b) found that the phonation type of lax vowels in the Zaiwa language is primarily modal voice with a slight breathy voice, while the phonation type of tense vowels is primarily creaky voice.

## Tense/lax voices in the Jingpo language

The Jingpo language has 31 initials, 88 finals and four tones (Liu, 1984). There are also five tense and five lax vowels in the Jingpo language. They are treated as different phonation types with the lax vowels being produced in modal voice and the tense vowels being produced in creaky voice (Kong, 2001b).

# Features of Phonation Types

To explore the voice features of different phonation types, a study was performed based on the analysis of EGG signals (Kong, 2001b). The speech materials were selected from the recordings of six languages collected in the aforementioned studies (Caodao & Kong, 1999; Kong, 1996, 1999, 2001b; Shen & Kong, 1999). These languages showed different phonation types: modal voice, creaky voice (with unstable F0), breathy voice, and fry voice (with relatively stable F0). We classified modal voice into three subcategories based on their acoustic features: high pitch, middle pitch and low pitch. High-pitched voice is different from falsetto. High-pitched voice has a relatively higher OQ and lower SQ when compared to the middle-pitch modal voice. In contrast, falsetto voice has an OQ of 100%. High-pitched voice is often used to convey phonemic meanings in some Chinese languages.

The results showed that fry voice had the lowest pitch (66.45 Hz), with an increasing pitch in the order of breathy voice, creaky voice, modal voice and high-pitched voice (261.21 Hz). Fry voice had the highest SQ (361.65), while breathy voice had the lowest (195.08). Fry voice also had the highest OQ (65.86), while creaky voice had the lowest (47.56).

# High-Speed Analysis of Phonation Types

High-speed analysis has been used to study the features of different phonation types (Kong, 2001b). A set of glottal measurements is extracted from the images (Kong, 2001b), which includes: (1) GA; (2) left GA; (3) right GA; (4) anterior GA; (5) posterior GA; (6) left glottal width; (7) right glottal width; (8) anterior glottal length; (9) posterior glottal length; (10) ratio of glottal length to glottal width; (11) F0; (12) OQ; and (13) SQ. Examples of modal, falsetto and creaky voice are described below, respectively.

## Modal voice

The montage and the glottal measurements in graphical format that represent a male modal voice are shown in Figure 15.4. A complete cycle of glottal vibration is illustrated, with the set of glottal measures drawn along the time axis. It is shown that the open phase roughly equals the close phase (OQ ≈ 50%), the opening phase roughly equals the closing phase (SQ ≈ 100%), and the vocal folds vibrate symmetrically in the left/right and anterior/posterior dimensions.

## Falsetto voice

Falsetto is a phonation type that enables a singer to sing notes beyond the vocal range of normal or modal voice to express strong emotion. This is not normally used in daily communication except in some individuals who have abnormal voice conditions or on some very rare occasions. Figure 15.5 demonstrates a female falsetto voice with 24 frames of glottal images. The glottis is constantly opened (OQ = 100%), and the vocal folds are vibrated with a small amplitude. The graph of the GA is presented as a sinusoid curve, which implies a strong low-frequency energy and high-frequency attenuation in spectrum. The opening phase is roughly the same as the closing phrase (SQ ≈ 100%).

## Creaky voice

Creaky voice is typically characterized by a low F0. In Mandarin Chinese, this often appears in the third lexical tone spoken by male individuals. From a physiological perspective, male speakers can produce creaky voice more easily than female speakers because the former have comparatively longer and thicker vocal folds.

A special case of male creaky voice is shown in Figure 15.6. The vocal folds are shortened, which leads to a relatively small GA. The existence of double-pulse and triple-pulse glottal waves is indicated in the graph of the GA. These may pose a big challenge to defining the concept of 'fundamental frequency' in the case of creaky voice.

# Concluding Remarks

Advances in the physiological and acoustic technologies have allowed researchers in China to expand and refine their research methodology in

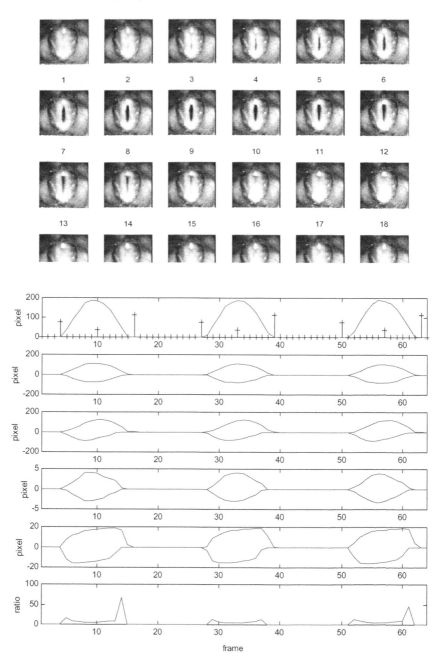

**Figure 15.4** High-speed images and extracted measures of a male modal voice
Notes: The six rows of graphs from the top downwards are: (1) full GA; (2) left and right half GA;
(3) anterior and posterior half GA; (4) left and right half glottal width; (5) anterior and posterior
half glottal length; (6) the ratio of glottal length to width, respectively.

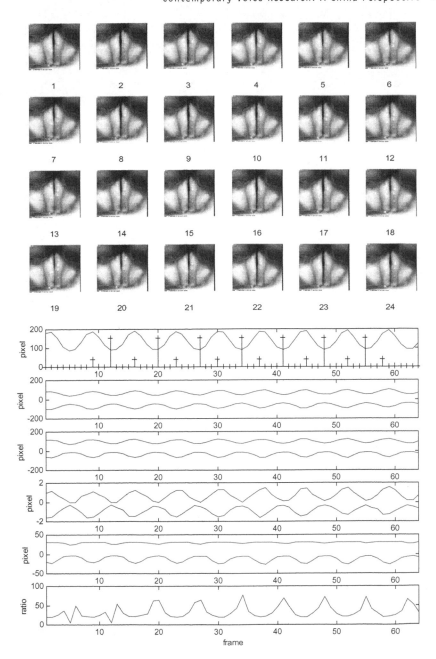

**Figure 15.5** High-speed images and extracted measures of glottis of a female falsetto voice

Notes: The six rows of graphs from the top downwards are: (1) full GA; (2) left and right half GA; (3) anterior and posterior half GA; (4) left and right half glottal width; (5) anterior and posterior half glottal length; (6) the ratio of glottal length to width, respectively.

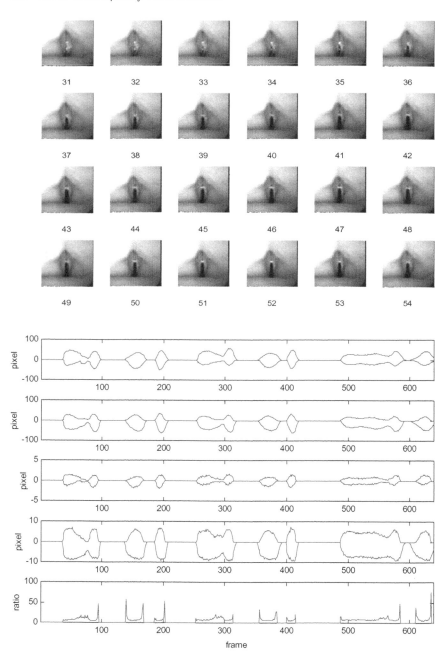

**Figure 15.6** High-speed images and extracted measures of glottis of a male fry voice
Notes: The six rows of graphs from the top downwards are: (1) full GA; (2) left and right half GA; (3) anterior and posterior half GA; (4) left and right half glottal width; (5) anterior and posterior half glottal length; (6) the ratio of glottal length to width, respectively.

voice science. The studies on voice characteristics in different phonation types in Chinese languages using these technologies have shed more light on the understanding of these phonation types.

In the field of phonetics and linguistics, researchers in China have benefited from the availability of new instrumentation. For example, the analysis of dynamic glottal images using high-speed laryngoscopy enables phoneticians/linguists to integrate a physiological model of vocal fold vibration into their phonetic/linguistic theories. This new knowledge of voice characteristics of different phonation types is not only useful for understanding the languages used by these different ethnic Chinese groups, but can also form the basis for possible further assessments and treatment protocols in the voice pathology and voice therapy areas.

## References

Alku, P. (1992) Glottal wave analysis with pitch synchronous iterative adaptive inverse filtering. *Speech Communication* 11 (2–3), 109–118.

Caodao, B. and Kong, J. (1999) EGG study of 84 Mongolian speakers. Paper presented at the the 4th National Conference on Modern Phonetics, Beijing.

Chang, H. (1986) *Overview of Lahu Language*. Beijing: Ethnic Publishing House. [常竑恩 (1986) 拉祜语简志 北京: 民族出版社.]

Chen, Z. and Lei, X. (1984) *Overview of Western Yugur Language*. Beijing: Ethnic Publishing House. [陈宗正, 雷选春(1984) 西部裕固语简志. 北京: 民族出版社.]

Childers, D.G., Hicks, D.M., Moore, G.P., Eskenazi, L. and Lalwani, A.L. (1990) Electroglottography and vocal fold physiology. *Journal of Speech and Hearing Research* 33 (2), 245–254.

Dao, B. (1983) *Overview of Mongolian Language*. Beijing: Ethnic Publishing House. [道布 (1983) 蒙古语简志. 北京: 民族出版社.]

Dickson, B.C., Esling, J.H. and Snell, R.C. (1994) Real-time processing of electroglottographic waveforms for the evaluation of phonation types. Paper presented at the Third International Conference on Spoken Language Processing (ICSLP 94), 18–22 September, Yokohama, Japan.

Fant, G. and Gauffin, J. (1994) *Speech Science and Technology Yan yu kexue yu yan yu jishu* (trans. J. Zhang). Beijing: Commercial Press.

Hall, K.D. and Yairi, E. (1992) Fundamental frequency, jitter, and shimmer in preschoolers who stutter. *Journal of Speech and Hearing Research* 35 (5), 1002–1008.

Holmberg, E.B., Hillman, R.E., Perkell, J.S., Guiod, P.C. and Goldman, S.L. (1995) Comparisons among aerodynamic, electroglottographic, and acoustic spectral measures of female voice. *Journal of Speech and Hearing Research* 38 (6), 1212–1223.

Horii, Y. (1985) Jitter and shimmer in sustained vocal fry phonation. *Folia Phoniatrica et Logopaedica* 37 (2), 81–86.

Kiritani, S., Hirose, H. and Imagawa, H. (1993) High-speed digital image analysis of vocal cord vibration in diplophonia. *Speech Communication* 13 (1–2), 23–32.

Kirk, P.L., Ladefoged, P. and Ladefoged, J. (1984) Using a spectrograph for measures of phonation types in a natural language. *UCLA Working Papers in Phonetics* 59, 102–113.

Kong, J. (1996) Hani yu fa sheng lei xing sheng xue yanjiu ji yin zhi gai nian de tao lun [Study on phonation types and timbre of Hani language]. *Min zu yu wen [Minority Languages of China]* 1, 40–46.

Kong, J. (1999) Correlation and classification study on EGG parameters of Mongolian. Paper presented at the 4th National Conference on Modern Phonetics, Beijing.

Kong, J. (2001a) *Correlation and Classification Study on EGG Parameters of Mandarin.* Beijing: Qin Hua University Press.

Kong, J. (2001b) *Lun yu yan fa sheng [On language phonation].* Bejing: Zhong yang min zu da xue chu ban she [Central University for Nationalities Press].

Kong, J. (2007) *Dynamic Laryngeal and Physiological Model.* Beijing: Peking University Press.

Kong, J.P. and Yiu, E.M-L. (2011) High speed laryngoscopy. In E.P.-M. Ma and E.M.-L. Yiu (eds) *Handbook of Clinical Voice Assessment.* San Diego, Plural Publishing.

Kong, J., Caodao, B., Chen, J. and Shen, M. (1997) Acoustic study of jitter, shimmer and tremors in Mandarin: Theory and application of signal processing. Paper presented at the Conference on Speech, Image and Communication Signal Processing of China (SICS 1997), Zhengzhou, China.

Ladefoged, P. (1973) The features of the larynx. *Journal of Phonetics* 1 (1), 73–83.

Ladefoged, P. (1988) Discussion of phonetics: A note on some terms for phonation types. In O. Fujimura (ed.) *Vocal Physiology: Voice Production, Mechanisms and Functions* (pp. 373–375). New York: Raven Press.

Ladefoged, P., Maddieson, I., Jackson, M. and Huffman, M. (1987) Characteristics of the voice source. Paper presented at the European Conference on Speech Technology (ECST-1987), Edinburgh.

Ladefoged, P., Maddieson, I. and Jackson, M. (1988) Investigating phonation types in different languages. In O. Fujimura (ed.) *Vocal Physiology: Voice Production, Mechanisms and Functions* (pp. 297–317). New York: Raven Press.

Laver, J. (1980) *The Phonetic Description of Voice Quality.* Cambridge: Cambridge University Press.

Li, Y. and Wang, E. (1986) *Overview of Hani Language.* Beijing: Ethnic Publishing House. [李永燧, 王尔松(1986) 哈尼语简志. 北京：民族出版社.]

Lindestad, P.A., Sodersten, M., Merker, B. and Granqvist, S. (2001) Voice source characteristics in Mongolian 'throat singing' studied with high-speed imaging technique, acoustic spectra, and inverse filtering. *Journal of Voice* 15 (1), 78–85.

Liu, L. (1984) *Overview of Jingpho Language Jingpo zu yu yan jian zhi (Jingpo yu).* Beijing: Ethnic Publishing House.

Maddieson, I. and Hess, S. (1986) 'Tense' and 'lax' revisited: More on phonation type and pitch in minority languages in China. *UCLA Working Papers in Phonetics* 63, 103–109.

Maddieson, I. and Ladefoged, P. (1985) 'Tense' and 'lax' in four minority languages of China. *UCLA Working Papers in Phonetics* 60, 59–83.

Orlikoff, R.F. (1991) Assessment of the dynamics of vocal fold contact from the electroglottogram: Data from normal male subjects. *Journal of Speech and Hearing Research* 34 (5), 1066–1072.

Rothenberg, M. and Mahshie, J.J. (1988) Monitoring vocal fold abduction through vocal fold contact area. *Journal of Speech and Hearing Research* 31 (3), 338–351.

Shen, M. and Kong, J. (1998) MDVP (multi-dimensional voice processing) study on sustained vowels of Mandarin through EGG signal. Paper presented at the Conference on Phonetics of the Languages in China, Hong Kong.

Shen, M. and Kong, J. (1999) Correlation and classification study on EGG parameters of Yi language. Paper presented at the 4th National Conference on Modern Phonetics, Beijing.

Sun, H. and Liu, L. (1986) *Overview of Nu language.* Beijing: Ethnic Publishing House. [孙宏开, 刘璐. (1986) 怒族语言简志. 北京：民族出版社.]

Thongkum, T.L. (1988) Phonation types in Mon-Khmer languages. In O. Funimura (ed.) *Voice Production: Mechanisms and Functions* (pp. 319–333). New York: Raven Press.

Traill, A. and Jackson, M. (1988) Speaker variation and phonation type in Tsonga nasals. *Journal of Phonetics* 16, 385–400.

Wang, F. (1985) *Overview of Miao Language.* Beijing: Ethnic Publishing House. [王辅世. (1985) 苗语简志. 北京：民族出版社.]

Wu, Z. (1981) Several features of the adjective in Axi Yi language. *Minority Languages of China* 3.

Xu, X. and Xu, G. (1984) *Overview of Zaiwa Language*. Beijing: Ethnic Publishing House. [徐悉艰, 徐桂珍. (1984) 景颇族语言简志 (载瓦语). 北京: 民族出版社.]

Xu, L. and Zhao, Y. (1984) *Overview of Bai Language*. Beijing: Ethnic Publishing House. [徐琳, 赵衍荪(1984) 白语简志 北京: 民族出版社.]

Xu, L., Mu, Y. and Gai, X. (1986) *Overview of Lisu Language*. Beijing: Ethnic Publishing House. [徐琳, 木玉璋, 盖兴之(1986) 傈僳简志 北京:民族出版社.]

Xuan, D., Jin, X. and Zhao, X. (1985) *Overview of Korean Language*. Beijing: Ethnic Publishing House. [宣德五, 金祥元, 赵习. (1985) 朝鲜语简志. 北京: 民族出版社.]

Yoshinaga, I. and Kong, J. (2011) Some phonatory characteristics of Tibetan Buddhist chants. *Journal of the Phonetic Society of Japan* 5 (2), 83–90.

Zhou, Z. and Yan, Q. (1984) *Overview of Wa Language*. Beijing: Ethnic Publishing House. [周植志, 颜其香. (1984) 佤语简志. 北京: 民族出版社].

# 16 Analysis of Professional Voice Users in the Clinical Setting

## Cate Madill and Patricia McCabe

In the last 10 years Australian researchers, speech pathologists and ear, nose and throat surgeons have conducted internationally recognised, high-quality research over a wide range of subject areas in voice. Dominant themes in the Australian research have been those of instrumental analysis of voice and the vocal characteristics of professional voice users. A range of studies have both utilised and developed instrumental assessments, specifically acoustic analysis and visual assessment of the vocal tract.

## Validity and Reliability of the Recorded Signal and Acoustic Analysis

Acoustic analysis is one of the most common instrumental measures used in assessing the vocal signal in both disordered and non-disordered voice populations. Australian researchers have used acoustic analysis to investigate a range of research questions and also focussed specifically on the utility, validity and reliability of acoustic analysis.

It is well documented that the equipment used, the recording environment, the recording protocols, speakers' characteristics and the type of analysis conducted on the signals can influence the validity and reliability of the results (e.g. Deliyski *et al.*, 2006). Recommendations to improve both the recording and analysis of voice samples by researchers and clinicians were provided by Vogel and Maruff (2008) and Vogel and Morgan (2009) following their investigations of various signal acquisition hardware and analysis processes. Vogel and Maruff (2008) reported that recordings captured with solid state, hard drive and standard laptop recorders are appropriate for acquiring samples for analysis for a selected range of acoustic measures including fundamental frequency (F0), the 1st and 2nd formants, and multi-dimensional voice profile analysis of absolute jitter, percent jitter, noise-to-harmonic ratio, pitch perturbation quotient, relative average perturbation, and shimmer in dB.

In both Vogel and Maruff (2008) and Vogel and Morgan (2009), strict recommendations for set-up of equipment, including configuration of microphones and recording devices, are provided. These recommendations should be routinely followed by speech pathologists to ensure the reliability of recording:

> the highest quality recording would be made by using a stand-alone hard disc recorder, an independent mixer to attenuate the incoming signal, and insulated wiring combined with a high quality microphone in an anechoic chamber or sound treated room. (Vogel & Morgan, 2009: 437)

The acoustic analysis of large numbers of voice recordings has previously proved difficult, given the time required to manually analyse each file. A process of large batch processing of voice files has been developed by Vogel *et al.* (2009b), who compared voice acoustic analysis results arising from manual categorisation and automated categorisation of 1120 voice files. The automated categorisation was conducted using a PRAAT script based around identification of F0. The results from the two methods for typical voices were statistically equivalent despite a huge difference in processing time required. Large batch processing of voice files was therefore thought to be a reliable approach to data acquisition. The authors suggested caution in applying the automated approach to disordered voices as some 'Individuals with frequency profiles outside expected levels may not be analysed accurately by using automated acoustic analysis' (Vogel *et al.*, 2009b: 323). However, 'sex-specific pitch settings' (Vogel *et al.*, 2009b: 323) were recommended to ensure that results are equivalent to the analysis of samples individually. This form of large-scale analysis creates new opportunities for the objective assessment of the voice in the theatre-voice and other voice training contexts.

Two acoustic measures of hypernasality were compared by Vogel *et al.* (2009a) in an effort to establish an alternative to the gold standard of perceptual judgement. Of the two measures examined (voice-high-tone-to-low-tone ratio; one-third octave spectra), only the one-third octave spectra was moderately reliable in separating disordered from non-disordered resonance.

Finally, Vogel *et al.* (2011) reported a series of five studies which systematically examined acoustic measures of timing and frequency as used with neurologically normal and impaired adults. These studies examined the reliability, stability (two studies) and sensitivity (two studies) of common measures of speech and voice performance, such as F0 and percent pause time, in sustained /a/, counting, recitation of days of the week, reading of the grandfather passage (Darley *et al.*, 1975) and free monologue, and the acoustic measures. Of 61 variables examined, 36 were stable over the medium term. This stability was found across various tasks. The greatest inter-task stability was found between trials two and three of five, which suggested that the initial and final trials might be less stable than median ones. Additionally, the researchers examined whether the stability was influenced by the Lombard effect and reported that frequency-based measures changed in response to background noise but timing-based measures did not. Timing measures generally reliably separated healthy and disordered participants across tasks.

# Professional Voice Users

Australian researchers have taken a particularly keen interest in the science of professional voice use and performers. Therefore, a number of studies have employed instrumentation to investigate the vocal function of professional voice users and performances.

## Acoustic measurement of the singing voice

There has been specific interest in the acoustic characteristics of the singing voice trained in the so-called classical style and the voices of opera singers. This style of singing requires distinct technical and performative features to meet the demands of the genre. Therefore, researchers have pursued a deeper understanding of these elements. Acoustic analysis of the energy characteristics in the spectrum using long term average spectrum (LTAS) analysis has been a specific focus of investigation into a range of singing phenomena. For example, the imperative of opera singers to be heard over an orchestra without amplification has been investigated using a range of studies that used acoustic analyses of the high spectral energy components, the so-called singer's formant or formant cluster (Sundberg, 2001). The high-frequency spectral energy in national and international standard soprano singers was compared across different song types, loudness levels and in different performance spaces (Barnes et al., 2004). Using the LTAS as the primary acoustic measure, this study found no evidence for a soprano singer's formant. There was evidence that high-frequency energy was more consistently present in singers performing regularly at international standard, and was typically present in all of the singers across vowel and song conditions.

Singing power ratio (SPR) and energy ratio (ER) based on LTAS analysis was used by Reid and colleagues (2007) to investigate whether there are acoustic differences between the voices of professional opera singers performing in chorus versus solo modes of singing. No significant differences were found between the overall power in the singers' formant or vibrato used in the two modes of singing. LTAS, SPR and ER have also been used to investigate the auditory-perceptual correlates of acoustic features in female classical singers (Kenny & Mitchell, 2006). However, no significant correlations between perceptual judgements and SPR and ER were found. An alternative method of calculating ER and SPR, the short-term energy ratio (STER) was developed to examine the effects of training in nine male classical singers (Ferguson et al., 2010). This form of calculation produced more detailed data and provided greater insight into the variety of strategies that these classical singers use at different levels of training to achieve increased energy in the high-frequency spectrum.

Both vibrato and *messa di voce* have been analysed using various LTAS, F0 and intensity in sound pressure level (SPL) measures including spectral balance (SB) and SPL linearity. Collyer *et al.* (2007) used SPL and analysis of linearity and symmetry of SB to analyse the *messa di voce* of trained female classical singers. Howes *et al.* (2004) used analysis of F0 to calculate vibrato rate and vibrato extent, which correlated moderately with expert auditory-perceptual judgements. LTAS and vibrato analysis were also used by Jacobs and Kenny (2005) to ascertain that the flexible fibre-optic laryngoscopy procedure did not affect the production and vocal quality of highly trained operatic singers. Noise measures such as harmonic-to-noise ratio have also been used to measure the performance effects on voices of choral tenors (Kitch *et al.*, 1996). However, no correlations between acoustic and auditory-perceptual judgements were found.

## Acoustic measurement of the spoken voice

The professional spoken voice, including student and professional actors and teachers, has also been of specific interest to Australian researchers. The effects of training on the voice have been evaluated using acoustic analysis in student actor and a range of professional voice users. These studies have demonstrated mixed effects of training across different voice training approaches and populations. Perturbation measures were observed to increase following 12 months of actor training (Walzak *et al.*, 2008). Conversely, a significant decrease in noise and perturbation measures was observed in voice recordings taken from professional voice users before and after training in differentiated vocal tract control and increased exertion during phonation (Bagnall & McCulloch, 2005).

Preliminary support for an actor's formant, similar to that of a singer's formant, was provided by Pinczower and Oates (2005), who observed increased acoustic energy in the higher part of the acoustic spectrum in maximally projected actors' voices. Pasa *et al.* (2007) used maximum phonation time (MPT) and maximum phonational frequency range (MPFR) to demonstrate the relative effectiveness of vocal hygiene training and vocal function exercises in preventing voice disorders in primary school teachers. Both narrow- and wide-band spectral analyses were utilised in analysing tonal F0 and laryngealisation to differentiate Vietnamese female teachers with and without muscle tension dysphonia (Nguyen & Kenny, 2009).

## Self-reported voice disorders in professional voice users

A small but influential subset of the professional voice users literature arises from researching into the prevalence of voice disorders in various professional voice user types. Self-reported voice problems in three groups of professional singers and a group of matched controls were examined by Phyland *et al.* (1999). Singers were more likely than non-singers to report voice disorders but no difference in voice disability was reported across the singer groups.

The self-reported prevalence of voice problems in Australian schoolteachers were examined by Russell and colleagues (1998), who found a 20% annual prevalence. These researchers followed up by demonstrating efficacy in addressing these problems through the use of a video training package (Oates & Russell, 1998). These results can be compared with the data collected from the self-report of voice disorders in the general population by Russell *et al.* (2005), in which the prevalence across the adult years was 6.8%.

## Visualisation of the Vocal Tract and Larynx

Visualisation of the larynx has been considered as a clinically essential instrumental voice assessment technique with greater objectivity than auditory-perceptual assessment. Australian researchers have made a substantial contribution to improving the reliability of rating visual images of the larynx and identifying the limitations and factors affecting laryngoscopic interpretation. Pemberton *et al.* (1993) developed a rating tool for nasendoscopic evaluation of a range of laryngeal parameters both at rest and during phonation, using both constant and stroboscopic light. The Australian Fiberscopic Profile demonstrated high inter-judge agreement with a videostroboscopic rating tool (Bless *et al.*, 1987). This rating tool was revised by Havas and Priestley (1993) to provide clearer definitions of specific laryngeal parameters and to enable more efficient and accurate reporting of the assessment. Madill *et al.* (2010) investigated the reliability of experienced speech pathologists rating nasendoscopic footages of trained speakers and found that raters were more reliable in *identifying* movements of laryngeal structures than *measuring* the amount of movement. Ratings of false vocal fold activity and larynx height changes were more reliable than ratings of true vocal fold closure and true vocal fold mass using nasendoscopy.

The effect of laryngeal nasendoscopy on the vocal performance of young adult females with normal voices was investigated by Lim *et al.* (1998). Maximum phonational frequency range was significantly reduced following nasal topical anaesthesia during the procedure. During the nasendoscopy procedure, maximum phonation time was reduced and speaking F0, minimum F0 when singing scales and ratings of breathiness by experienced listeners were all increased. Children's perception of discomfort and pain when undergoing nasendoscopy for investigation of voice and resonance disorders was also investigated by Hay *et al.* (2009). This study found that children aged between 4 and 18 years, on average, perceived the procedure to be moderately painful, with children aged 4–7 years old reporting significantly more pain than children aged 8–18 years.

# Electroglottograph

The electrogolottograph (EGG), also known as the laryngograph, is an instrumental voice measurement tool that has been used predominantly in the context of voice research, rather than standard clinical evaluation of the voice. It provides information on true vocal fold vibratory patterns, specifically information on F0, open and closed phases of the glottal cycle and is considered an indirect measure of true vocal fold contact during phonation. This tool has been used by Australian researchers in conjunction with acoustic analysis in investigations of the voice characteristics of chronic cough (CC) and paradoxical vocal fold movement (PVFM) (Vertigan *et al.*, 2008a). Individuals with CC/PVFM were found to have increased jitter, reduced harmonic-to-noise ratio and shorter closed phase of true vocal fold vibration. The outcomes of two treatments of chronic cough (Vertigan *et al.*, 2008b) were also evaluated using EGG and acoustic measures. EGG has also been used to investigate the effect of age and gender on true vocal fold vibrations (Ma & Love, 2010). This study revealed reduced true vocal fold contact in older versus younger males and increased vocal fold contact for older versus younger females. The authors also noted a significant effect of the phonation task on EGG measures, specifically suggesting that EGG measures obtained from connected speech samples are more accurate than those collected from prolonged vowel samples.

Australian researchers continue to contribute to global voice research in many areas of voice other than those discussed above. Technological advances and new instrumentation such as high-speed video-laryngoscopy and cepstral peak analyses pose further opportunities to discover even more about how the voice works, whether it is in the context of the disordered voice or in the vocal skill and demands of professional voice users. With research centres in many university and hospital settings, the future looks bright for Australian researchers to continue to contribute internationally to the knowledge base of voice science and the clinical management of professional voice users.

## References

Bagnall, A.D. and McCulloch, K. (2005) The impact of specific exertion on the efficiency and ease of the voice: A pilot study. *Journal of Voice* 19 (3), 384–390.

Barnes, J., Davis, P., Oates, J. and Chapman, J. (2004) The relationship between professional operatic soprano voice and high range spectral energy. *Journal of the Acoustical Society of America* 116, 530–538.

Bless, D. M., Hirano, M. and Feder, R. (1987) Videostroboscopic evaluation of the larynx. *Ear, Nose, & Throat Journal* 66 (7), 289–296.

Collyer, S., Davis, P., Thorpe, W. and Callaghan, J. (2007) Sound pressure level and spectral balance linearity and symmetry in the messa di voce of female classical singers. *Journal of the Acoustical Society of America* 121 (3), 1728–1736.

Darley, F.L., Aronson, A.E. and Brown, J.R. (1975) *Motor Speech Disorders*. Philadelphia: W.B. Saunders.

Deliyski, D.D., Shaw, H.S., Evans, M.K. and Vesselinov, R. (2006) Regression tree approach to studying factors influencing acoustic voice analysis. *Folia Phoniatrica et Logopaedica* 58, 274–288

Ferguson, S., Kenny, D.T. and Cabrera, D. (2010) Effects of training on time-varying spectral energy and sound pressure level in nine male classical singers. Effects of training on time-varying spectral energy and sound pressure level in nine male classical singers. *Journal of Voice* 24, 39–46.

Havas, T. and Priestley, J. (1993) The revised Australian fiberscopic profile. *Journal of Voice* 7, 377–381.

Hay, I., Oates, J., Giannini, A., Berkowitz, R. and Rotenberg, B. (2009) Pain perception of children undergoing nasendoscopy for investigation of voice and resonance disorders. *Journal of Voice* 23, 380–388.

Howes, P., Callaghan, J., Davis, P., Kenny, D. and Thorpe, W. (2004) The relationship between measured vibrato characteristics and perception in Western operatic singing. *Journal of Voice* 18 (2), 216–230.

Jacobs, M.A. and Kenny, D.T. (2005) Effects of topical anesthetic and flexible fiberoptic laryngoscopy on professional sopranos. *Journal of Voice* 19 (4), 645–664.

Kenny, D.T. and Mitchell, H.F. (2006) Acoustic and perceptual appraisal of vocal gestures in the female classical voice. *Journal of Voice* 20, 55–70.

Kitch, J.A., Oates, J. and Greenwood, K. (1996) Performance effects on the voices of 10 choral tenors: Acoustic and perceptual findings. *Journal of Voice* 10 (3), 217–227.

Lim, V.P.C., Oates, J.M., Phyland, D.J. and Campbell, M.J. (1998) Effects of laryngeal endoscopy on the vocal performance of young adult females with normal voices. *Journal of Voice* 12, 68–77.

Ma, E.P.-M. and Love, A.L. (2010) Electroglottographic evaluation of age and gender effects during sustained phonation and connected speech. *Journal of Voice* 24 (2), 146–152.

Madill, C., Sheard, C. and Heard, R. (2010) Differentiated vocal tract control and the reliability of interpretations of nasendoscopic assessment. *Journal of Voice* 24 (3), 337–345.

Nguyen, D.D. and Kenny, D.T. (2009) Effects of muscle tension dysphonia on tone phonation: Acoustic and perceptual studies in Vietnamese female teachers. *Journal of Voice* 23 (4), 446–459.

Oates, J.M. and Russell, A. (1998) Learning voice analysis using an interactive multimedia package: Development and preliminary evaluation. *Journal of Voice* 12 (4), 500–512.

Pasa, G., Oates, J. and Dacakis, G. (2007) The relative effectiveness of vocal hygiene training and vocal function exercises in preventing voice disorders in primary school teachers. *Logopedics Phoniatrics Vocology* 32 (3), 128–140.

Pemberton, C., Russell, A., Priestley, J., Havas, T., Hooper, J. and Clark, P. (1993) Characteristics of normal larynges under flexible fiberscopic and stroboscopic examination: An Australian perspective. *Journal of Voice* 7 (4), 382–389.

Phyland, D.J., Oates, J.M. and Greenwood, K.M. (1999) Self-reported voice problems among three groups of professional singers. *Journal of Voice* 13 (4), 602–611.

Pinczower, R. and Oates, J. (2005) Vocal projection in actors: The long-term average spectral features that distinguish comfortable acting from voicing with maximal projection in male actors. *Journal of Voice* 19 (3), 440–453.

Reid, K., Davis, P., Oates, J., Carbrera, D., Ternström, S., Black, M., *et al.* (2007) The acoustic characteristics of professional opera singers performing in chorus versus solo mode. *Journal of Voice* 21, 35–45.

Russell, A., Oates, J.M. and Greenwood, K. (1998) Prevalence of voice problems in teachers. *Journal of Voice* 12 (4), 467–479.

Russell, A., Oates, J. and Greenwood, K. (2005) Prevalence of self-reported voice problems in the general population in South Australia. *International Journal of Speech-Language Pathology* 7, 24–30.

Sundberg, J. (2001) Level and center frequency of the singer's formant. *Journal of Voice* 15 (2), 176–186.

Vertigan, A.E., Theodoros, D.G., Winkworth, A.L. and Gibson, P.G. (2008a) Acoustic and electroglottographic voice characteristics in chronic cough and paradoxical vocal fold movement. *Folia Phoniatrica et Logopaedica* 60 (4), 210–216.

Vertigan, A.E., Theodoros, D.G., Winkworth, A.L. and Gibson, P.G. (2008b) A comparison of two approaches to the treatment of chronic cough: Perceptual, acoustic, and electroglottographic outcomes. *Journal of Voice* 22 (5), 581–589.

Vogel, A.P. and Maruff, P. (2008) Comparison of voice acquisition methodologies in speech research. *Behavior Research Methods* 40 (4), 982–987.

Vogel, A.P. and Morgan, A.T. (2009) Factors affecting the quality of sound recording for speech and voice analysis. *International Journal of Speech-Language Pathology* 11 (6), 431–437.

Vogel, A.P., Ibrahim, H.M., Reilly, S. and Kilpatrick, N. (2009a) A comparative study of two acoustic measures of hypernasality. *Journal of Speech, Language, and Hearing Research* 52, 1640–1651.

Vogel, A.P., Maruff, P., Snyder, P.J. and Mundt, J.C. (2009b) Standardization of pitch-range settings in voice acoustic analysis. *Behavior Research Methods* 41 (2), 318–324.

Vogel, A.P., Fletcher, J. Snyder, P.J., Fredrickson, A. and Maruff, P. (2011) Reliability, stability, and sensitivity to change and impairment in acoustic measures of timing and frequency. *Journal of Voice* 25 (2), 137–149.

Walzak, P., McCabe, P., Madill, C. and Sheard, C. (2008) Acoustic changes in student actors' voices after 12 months of training. *Journal of Voice* 22 (3), 300–313.

# 17 Contemporary Voice Research: A Belgian Perspective

## Marc De Bodt and Youri Maryn

## Objective Voice Measurements

The use of objective voice measurements in daily clinical practice entailed the need for a reliable and objective correlate for voice quality. Voice quality is described by Titze (1994) as a poorly defined term 'that includes all the leftover perceptions after pitch, loudness and phonetic category have been identified'. Consequently, since voice quality is everything except pitch, loudness and phonetic category, it includes all perceptual dimensions of the spectral envelope and its changes in time (Kreiman & Gerratt, 1998). As such, voice quality is a multidimensional perceptual construct in contrast to pitch, loudness and the voiced phonemes that are predominantly monodimensional (i.e. for which there are the single acoustic correlates fundamental frequency, intensity and formant frequency, respectively). Since voice quality is auditory-perceptual by nature (Shrivastav, 2003), its primary measurement technique is the auditory-perceptual rating scale. Standardized used protocols for the perceptual evaluation of voice and voice quality, such as the Grade, Roughness, Breathiness, Asthenicity and Strain scale (GRBAS) and the Consensus Auditory-Perceptual Evaluation of Voice (CAPE-V), have been presented respectively by Hirano (1981) and Kempster *et al.* (2009) and are commonly implemented in clinical voice assessment. However, because voice quality is an attribute of the acoustic wave emanating from the vocal tract of the speaker, numerous acoustic measuring techniques have been proposed as objective correlates of the perceptual ratings. Popular acoustic methods in voice quality assessment are vocal perturbation measures (e.g. jitter), and various ratios (e.g. noise-to-harmonics ratio).

The relationship between perceptual judgment and acoustic metrics has been studied by many investigators. Most studies have reported the quantitative correlation between isolated acoustic variables (e.g. jitter, shimmer, harmonics-to-noise ratio) with the perceptual judgment. An extensive overview of acoustic measurements related to voice quality can be found in Buder (2000). Furthermore, Maryn *et al.* (2009b) performed a meta-analysis on the correlations between auditory-perceptual evaluations and acoustic measures of overall voice quality. This meta-analysis revealed multiple-study based moderate to strong correlations with overall voice quality ratings for only six acoustic markers (out of possible 69 acoustic measures on sustained vowels and 26 acoustic measures on continuous speech). Maryn *et al.* (2009b) warned that, although acoustic measures are routinely utilized in clinical voice examinations, the results of their meta-analysis suggested that caution is warranted regarding the concurrent validity and thus the clinical utility of many of these measures. Buder (2000) suggested that it is probable that multivariate (and multitask) methods are needed for measuring vocal quality.

In order to overcome the limited predictive power of single acoustic markers and also motivated by the multidimensionality of voice, several researchers have advocated a multivariable approach for the prediction of voice quality and/or the discrimination between different perceptual categories and levels of dysphonia severity (Awan & Roy, 2006; Bhuta *et al.*, 2004; Eskenazi *et al.*, 1990; Giovanni *et al.*, 1996; Ma & Yiu, 2006; Maryn *et al.*, 2009a, 2010a; Piccirillo *et al.*, 1998; Wolfe *et al.*, 1995, 1997; Wuyts *et al.*, 2000; Yu *et al.*, 2001). Table 17.1 summarizes relevant methodological items and the most salient outcomes of these multivariate approaches.

Belgian research contributed considerably to the development of multivariate approaches and reflects the historical evolution from a monodimensional approach to a more refined multivariate- and multitask-based approach. The studies initially founded on sustained vowels only (Wuyts *et al.*, 2000) and later on both sustained vowels and connected speech (Maryn *et al.*, 2010a, 2010b).

# The Dysphonia Severity Index

The Dysphonia Severity Index (DSI) is based on a large multicenter database of voice patients and controls, constructed for the Belgian Study Group on Voice Disorders (Wuyts *et al.*, 1996). Data from a group of 387 adults between 8 and 80 years (53% female, 47% male) were used for the calculation of the DSI. Among the subjects were 68 healthy controls (43 women, 25 men), recruited at random in the participating centers. A group of 319 dysphonic patients was included. The assessment included history and clinical antecedents, stroboscopic evaluation, perceptual assessment (GRBAS), acoustic analysis (Multidimensional Voice Program (MDVP)), voice range profile, aerodynamic measurements (e.g. maximum phonation time, vital capacity) and self-rating. The methods are described in detail elsewhere (Wuyts *et al.*, 2000).

**Table 17.1** Methods and results of multivariable approaches in the objective measurement of overall voice quality

| Source | Number of subjects | Multivariate statistical method | Speech task[a] | Objective measures included in multivariate model | Perceptual evaluation of overall voice quality | | Results | |
|---|---|---|---|---|---|---|---|---|
| | | | | | Dimension | Scale | Absolute correlation | Classification accuracy[b] |
| Eskenazi et al. (1990) | 16 | Multiple linear regression analysis | SV – 2 s [i.] | • Pitch amplitude<br>• Harmonics-to-noise ratio | Overall severity | EAI 7 points | 0.75 | – |
| Wolfe et al. (1995) | 80 | Stepwise multiple regression analysis | SV – 1 s [a.] | • Relative average perturbation<br>• Fundamental frequency | Quality of phonation | EAI 7 points | 0.56 | – |
| Giovanni et al. (1996) | 245 | Direct-entry discriminant function analysis | SV – 2 s [a.] | • Percent jitter<br>• Corrected spectrum<br>• Ratio of oral airflow to intensity (glottal leakage)<br>• Duration of the attack period | G, grade | EAI 5 points | – | 66.1% correct |
| Wolfe et al. (1997) | 51 | Multiple regression analysis | SV – 1 s [a.] and [i.] | • Noise-to-harmonics ratio<br>• Standard deviation of fundamental frequency, Percent jitter, Relative average perturbation or Pitch perturbation quotient | Severity of dysphonia | EAI 7 points | 0.61 | – |

(continued)

**Table 17.1** (*Continued*) Methods and results of multivariable approaches in the objective measurement of overall voice quality

| Source | Number of subjects | Multivariate statistical method | Speech task[a] | Objective measures included in multivariate model | Perceptual evaluation of overall voice quality | | Results | |
|---|---|---|---|---|---|---|---|---|
| | | | | | Dimension | Scale | Absolute correlation | Classification accuracy[b] |
| Wolfe et al. (1997) | 51 | Multiple regression analysis | SV – 1 s [a.] and [i.] | • Noise-to-harmonics ratio<br>• Percent shimmer, Shimmer in dB or Amplitude perturbation quotient | Severity of dysphonia | EAI 7 points | 0.63 | – |
| Piccirillo et al. (1998) | 33 | Logistic regression analysis | SV for MPT, VRP, etc. | • Subglottic pressure<br>• Airflow at lips<br>• Fundamental frequency range<br>• Maximum phonation time | G, grade | EAI 4 points | 0.58 | – |
| Wuyts et al. (2000) | 387 | Stepwise logistic regression analysis | SV for MPT, VRP, etc. | • Maximum phonation time<br>• Highest fundamental frequency<br>• Softest intensity<br>• Percent jitter | G, grade | EAI 4 points | – | 49.9% correct |

| | | | | | | | | |
|---|---|---|---|---|---|---|---|---|
| Yu et al. (2001) | 84 | Stepwise discriminant function analysis | SV – 2 s [a. SV for VRP] | • Fundamental frequency range<br>• Fundamental frequency<br>• Lyapunov coefficient<br>• Maximum phonation time<br>• Estimated subglottic pressure<br>• Total signal-to-noise ratio | G, grade | EAI 4 points | – | 86.0% correct |
| Bhuta et al. (2004) | 37 | Stepwise multiple regression analysis | SV – 3 s [a.] | • Voice turbulence index<br>• Noise-to-harmonics ratio<br>• Soft phonation index | G, grade | EAI 4 points | 0.66 | – |
| Awan & Roy (2006) | 134 | Stepwise multiple regression analysis | SV – 1 s [a.] | • Ratio of the amplitude of the cepstral peak prominence to the expected amplitude of the cepstral peak<br>• Discrete Fourier transform ratio $(energy_{<4000Hz} / energy_{>4000\,Hz})$<br>• Logarithm of shimmer<br>• Inverse square root of the pitch sigma | Severity of dysphonia | EAI 7 points | 0.88 | – |

(continued)

**Table 17.1** (*Continued*) Methods and results of multivariable approaches in the objective measurement of overall voice quality

| Source | Number of subjects | Multivariate statistical method | Speech task[a] | Objective measures included in multivariate model | Perceptual evaluation of overall voice quality | | Results | |
| --- | --- | --- | --- | --- | --- | --- | --- | --- |
| | | | | | Dimension | Scale | Absolute correlation | Classification accuracy[b] |
| Ma & Yiu (2006) | 153 | Direct-entry discriminant function analysis | SV for MPT, VRP, etc. | • Maximum phonation time <br> • Peak intraoral pressure <br> • Voice range profile area <br> • Relative amplitude perturbation | G, grade | EAI 11 points | – | 67.3% correct |
| Maryn et al. (2010a) | 251 | Stepwise multiple regression analysis | SV – 3 s [a.] <br> CS – 2 sentences | • Smoothed cepstral peak prominence <br> • Harmonics-to-noise ratio <br> • Shimmer local <br> • Shimmer local dB <br> • Slope of LTAS <br> • Tilt of trendline through LTAS | G, grade | EAI 4 points | 0.78 | 0.90 $A_{ROC}$ |
| Maryn et al. (2009a) | 16 (tracheo-esophageal voice) | Stepwise multiple regression analysis | SV – 3 s [a.] <br> CS – 2 sentences | • Cepstral peak prominence <br> • Mean height of second harmonic | G, grade | Paired comparison paradigm | 0.87 | – |

Notes: [a] SV, sustained vowel; CS, continuous speech; MPT, maximum phonation time; VRP, voice range profile.
[b] $A_{ROC}$, area under the ROC curve.

An initial univariate analysis of the relationship between GRBAS dimensions and acoustic measures revealed quite disappointing correlations. Wuyts *et al.* (1996) showed that the best Spearman's rank correlation between acoustic variables from the MDVP (Kay Elemetrics) and the GRBAS score in a large group of subjects ($N = 494$) did not exceed 0.53 for any of the GRBAS scale items. Although a lot of these correlations were statistically significant ($p < 0.001$), it was not possible to draw clinically useful conclusions about voice quality based on single variables that exhibit such low correlations with the perceived voice quality.

A multiparametric approach (stepwise logistic regression procedure) was then attempted to calculate an objective measure for voice quality. The variables used for the statistical analysis consisted of jitter (%), shimmer (%), noise-to-harmonic ratio (NHR), highest fundamental frequency (F0-High, Hz), lowest fundamental frequency (F0-Low, Hz), fundamental frequency range (F0-range, Hz), semitone range (ST-range), highest intensity (I-High, dB), lowest intensity (I-Low, dB), intensity range (I-range, dB), maximum phonation time (MPT, sec), vital capacity (VC, cc), phonation quotient (PQ, cc/sec), and the G (Grade from the GRBAS scale) score.

The DSI, being the discriminating rule calculated by the stepwise logistic regression, consists of a linear combination of four variables (the choice of variables in the DSI is entirely determined by the stepwise logistic regression procedure), where each variable has a different weight. The equation is:

$$DSI = 0.13 \times MPT \text{ (sec)} + 0.0053 \times F0\text{-High (Hz)} - 0.26 \times I\text{-Low (dB)}$$
$$-1.18 \times jitter \text{ (\%)} + 12.4$$

This DSI is the weighted combination of variables that reflects best the degree of hoarseness as expressed by the G from the GRBAS scale. The relation between G and the DSI as calculated in this first concept is represented by the linear regression (–●–) in Figure 17.1. The more negative this DSI is for a patient, the worse his or her vocal quality. The more positive it is, the better the vocal quality is. The initial regression-generated coefficients were post hoc multiplied with a scale factor in order to construct a practical scale where +5 corresponds to the average DSI of the G0 group and –5 to the average DSI of the G3 group. Table 17.2 lists the DSI values after scaling for the different G scores. Measurement errors on the individual components of the DSI inevitably give rise to an error on the final outcome measure. The calculated error of the DSI was 0.64, based on an average standard deviation of 1.6 sec for MPT, 39 Hz for F0-High, 1.7 dB(A) for I-Low, and 0.3% for jitter.

The gender effect is canceled out because of the opposite behavior of the MPT and F0-High for female and male subjects. The highest frequency (F0-High) is higher in females than in males but, on the other hand, MPT is longer in males than in females. Inclusion of both measurements in the index neutralizes the gender effect, so only one version of the DSI needs to be used for both sexes.

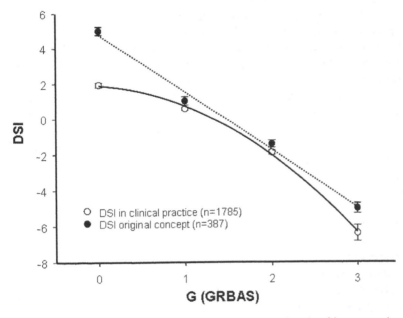

**Figure 17.1** Dysphonia Severity Index (DSI) versus G (grade of hoarseness)

The Pearson's correlation coefficient of the relation between DSI and VHI is $-0.79$ ($p < 0.001$). The DSI was transformed in such a way that, for the group of voices characterized by a G0, the DSI corresponds to $+5$, and for those patients with a G3 it corresponds to $-5$. The more negative this DSI is for a patient, the more his or her voice can be regarded as dysphonic. The higher it is, the better is his or her vocal quality. However, the DSI is not only limited to the interval $+5$, $-5$. In our clinical practice we sometimes obtain values of $-6$ and $+6$ and more. In extreme cases, the user should be aware of certain restrictions concerning the non-periodicity of some pathologic voice samples, as reported by Titze (1995).

It takes 10–15 min to collect the clinical measures (MPT, etc.) from a patient and to calculate the index using the above-mentioned equation. For this calculation a desktop calculator or spreadsheet is sufficient. Additionally,

**Table 17.2** Average Dysphonia Severity Index (DSI) values and standard errors for each grade (G) score

| G score | DSI ± standard error of the mean |
| --- | --- |
| $G_0$ | $5.00 \pm 0.23$ |
| $G_1$ | $1.02 \pm 0.25$ |
| $G_2$ | $-1.4 \pm 0.3$ |
| $G_3$ | $-5.0 \pm 0.8$ |

the use of anchor points of −5 and +5 facilitate the clinical use of the DSI. These aspects contribute largely to the ease of use of the DSI.

Additionally, we want to address the content and criterion validity of the DSI. Content validity refers to whether the index measures what it is intended to – that is, the degree of dysphonia. The four variables used in the DSI are individually all clear indicators of dysphonia, because their averages are significantly different for patients with vocal pathology as opposed to normal subjects (Wuyts et al., 1996). Additionally, the selection of these variables is based on a statistical stepwise procedure that constructs a rule to classify voices that are characterized by the scores G0–G3, which in turn represents the degree of dysphonia as perceived by the voice specialist. Considering these facts, it seems reasonable that the DSI meets the criteria of content validity.

Criterion validity refers to the accuracy of the DSI. How does it compare to a 'gold standard'? Auditory-perceptual judgments are typically the final arbiter in clinical decision-making and often provide the standards against which instrumental measures are evaluated (Kent, 1996). Inherently, the construction of the DSI is based on such a standard, being the Grade of the widely used perceptual GRBAS scale. To compare the DSI with an external measure, we correlated the DSI with the Voice Handicap Index. The high correlation between both measures adds to the criterion validity of the DSI. Moreover, this high correlation indicates that the DSI reflects not only the vocal quality of the patient but also reflects to a great extent the handicap as perceived by the patient.

The DSI has been used in daily practice now for more than 10 years. In order to evaluate how consistent the DSI is with the original concept, another 1765 cases were analyzed. The relation DSI_G for daily clinical practice is expressed in Figure 17.1 to be the –○– line. This demonstrates that the DSI is quite consistent, except for G0 cases corresponding more to DSI 2 than DSI 5. This may be explained by noting that, in clinical practice, healthy cases are rare and G0 is attributed to patients with a rather good but not excellent voice.

Hakkesteegt and colleagues (2006, 2008a, b, 2010) conducted a number of independent studies on the DSI. They investigated the influence of age and gender on the DSI in 118 controls and found no significant differences between males and females. Age, on the other hand, has a significant effect on the DSI for both sexes: the DSI decreases with advancing age.

The relation between DSI and overall severity G was investigated in 294 patients and in 118 controls. A high G-score corresponded with a low DSI. They determined the cut-off score where the DSI discriminates between patients and controls on 3. Furthermore they found that there was a high intra-subject reproducibility and a low inter-observer variability and that the DSI is applicable in evaluating the effects of voice therapy and phonosurgery. These independent studies and the recommendations of the authors underline the strengths of the DSI concept over a long period.

# The Acoustic Voice Quality Index

One of the major limitations of the DSI, however, was that the voice samples on which it is based are restricted to sustained vowels. Since sustained mid-vowel samples are relatively time-invariant, they can be elicited and produced comparatively easily in a standardized manner, and are not influenced by speech rate, stress, phonetic context or vocal pauses; acoustic analysis is possible with confounding complications. On the other hand, relying solely on a sustained vowel does not render the most ecologically valid voice assessment, one that truly reflects daily speech and voice use patterns (Maryn et al., 2010a). Consequently, the implementation of connected speech in the objective assessment of voice quality has attracted researchers' interest as it poses a new challenge.

To take into account these two types of speech stimuli (sustained vowel and connected speech) in the acoustic measurement of dysphonia severity, Maryn and colleagues started recording the first two sentences of a standardized Dutch text and the three medial seconds of a sustained /a/. Both recordings were then concatenated to one single sample, auditory-perceptually evaluated by five experienced listeners, and analyzed with 13 acoustic measures. The methods of their experiments have been described in detail elsewhere (Maryn et al., 2010a, 2010b). In the first experiment, voice samples from 251 normophonic and vocally disordered subjects were recorded (Maryn et al., 2010a). The Spearman rank-order correlations ($r_s$) between the acoustic measures and the mean G ratings revealed that the smoothed cepstral peak prominence (CPPs) best predicted the mean grade of dysphonia (G), followed by harmonics-to-noise ratio (HNR), cepstral peak prominence (CPP) and three shimmer measures (see Table 17.1). The other measures did not reach the level of $r_s = 0.60$. Furthermore, stepwise linear regression analysis with the 13 acoustic measures as independent variables revealed that a weighted combination of six acoustic metrics best parameterized the dysphonia severity of the concatenated voice recordings. Analogous to the DSI, this multivariate model was called the Acoustic Voice Quality Index (AVQI). The initial equation, based on the unstandardized coefficients of the regression, resulted in outcomes ranging from −0.39 to 3.50. However, for practical reasons and clinical feasibility, the equation was linearly rescaled to produce values on a scale from 0 to 10: AVQI = (3.295 − 0.111 × CPPs − 0.073 × HNR − 0.213 × shimmer local + 2.789 × shimmer local dB − 0.032 × slope + 0.077 × tilt) × 2.571. The initial $r_s$ between AVQI and mean G was 0.78, indicating strong concurrent validity for the group of 251 subjects. The coefficient of determination (i.e. $r_s^2$) was 0.61, denoting that 61% of mean G's variance is accounted for by AVQI (see Figure 17.2; Maryn et al., 2010a). Additional studies on the validity of the AVQI as an objective dysphonia severity measure revealed reasonable outcomes in terms of diagnostic accuracy and responsiveness to change (Maryn et al., 2010a, b).

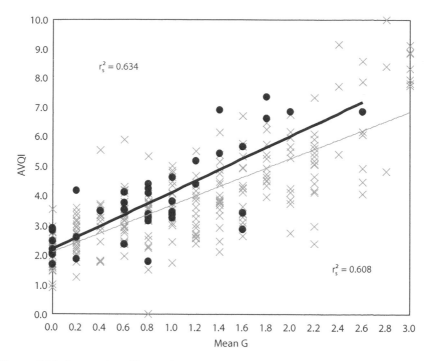

**Figure 17.2** Scatterplots illustrating Acoustic Voice Quality Index concurrent validity as an objective measure of dysphonia severity
Notes: The grey crossed scatters and regression line represent the 251 subjects from the first experiment (Maryn *et al.*, 2009b). The black circled scatters and regression line correspond with 39 subjects from the second experiment (Maryn *et al.*, 2010b).

In summary, the assessment of dysphonia severity and tracking of treatment outcomes ideally employ methods which examine both sustained vowels and continuous speech. To our knowledge, Maryn *et al.* (2010a, 2010b) were the first to build a multivariable model based on acoustic measures derived from both sustained vowels and connected speech. This 'Acoustic Voice Quality Index' implemented the medial 3 seconds of a sustained /a/ and the first two sentences of a phonetically balanced Dutch text and concatenated them into one single sound file, upon which six acoustic metrics were calculated. Measures of harmonic versus noise energy (HNR) and spectral talus (tilt and slope of the long-term average spectrum LTAS) have classically been associated with insufficient glottal closure and breathiness. Measures of amplitude perturbation (shimmer local and shimmer local dB) have traditionally been related to vibration irregularity and roughness. Although cepstral measures (CPPs) have mainly been associated with breathiness and less with roughness, it is hypothesized that all factors inflicting disruptions in the voice signal reduce the prominence of the first 'rahmonic'

(Ferrer *et al.*, 2007). Consequently, the AVQI combination includes different measures responsive to potential vibratory distortions at the level of the vocal folds, and thus serves as a measure of overall dysphonia severity.

Details of the validation process can be found in Maryn *et al.* (2010a, 2010b). These establish the robustness of the AVQI as a clinical measure of dysphonia severity, support its external validity and underscore its role as a valid treatment outcome measure in voice. Furthermore, because the AVQI can be determined using the freely available computer programs Praat and SpeechTool, it has the extra cachet of being accessible and affordable. In summary, as clinical management and government require objective evidence regarding treatment outcomes, the results of these experiments highlight that the AVQI merits special attention as a promising objective voice treatment outcomes measure.

# Conclusion

Overall voice quality has played an important role in Belgian voice research. Inaugurated by clinical events and the need for quantity-based decision-making, the development of the DSI and the AVQI reflects a clear evolution in the way dysphonia severity may be objectified using multiparametric approaches. Both indices have been constructed with perceptual 'Grade' as a criterion. Furthermore, both the DSI and the AVQI have been modeled on data pertaining to large and clinically representative groups of normophonic and dysphonic subjects. However, because of differing content, they reflect overall voice quality and dysphonia differently. Next to a comfortable sustained vowel for jitter, the DSI is based on performance-related tasks and challenged vowel productions for the voice range profile and the maximum phonation time. Because of the more challenging phonatory tasks, patients have to perform more and exhibit more of their vocal capacities for the DSI than for the AVQI, for which the acoustic analysis is limited to comfortable production of sustained vowels and connected speech without maximum performance. Consequently, the DSI is assumed to reflect better the limitations in vocal functioning, whereas the AVQI is hypothesized to correspond more explicitly with voice quality as distracted from real representative voice samples. As such, a complementary use of the two indices (i.e. the DSI as a more global measure of vocal functioning and voice disorder, and the AVQI as a measure specifically pertaining to overall voice quality) is expected to optimize objective voice assessment.

Finally, several future directions of Belgian research regarding clinical voice assessment can be mentioned here. Firstly, the complementary character of the DSI and the AVQI, and especially the degree with which their outcome is related to patient-perceived quality of life and quality of voice estimates, should further be investigated. Secondly, to increase the representativeness of objective voice quality assessment, it would be interesting to experiment with expanded portions of continuous speech in the AVQI. Third, because of phonetic differences between languages or dialects, it can be hypothesized that the implementation of continuous speech causes inter-language or interdialect differences. Therefore, a multi-linguistic investigation and if possible a cross-linguistic validation of the AVQI is warranted if it is to be promoted as a more universal metric of dysphonia severity.

## References

Awan, S.N. and Roy, N. (2006) Toward the development of an objective index of dysphonia severity: A four factor acoustic model. *Clinical Linguistics & Phonetics* 20 (1), 35–49.

Bhuta, T., Patrick, L. and Garnett, J.D. (2004) Perceptual evaluation of voice quality and its correlation with acoustic measurements. *Journal of Voice* 18 (3), 299–304.

Buder, E.H. (2000) Acoustic analysis of voice quality: A tabulation of algorithms 1902–1990. In R.D. Kent and M.J. Ball (eds) *Voice Quality Measurement* (pp. 119–244). San Diego: Singular Publishing.

Eskenazi, L., Childers, D.G. and Hicks, D.M. (1990) Acoustic correlates of vocal quality. *Journal of Speech and Hearing Research* 33 (2), 298–306.

Ferrer, C.A., De Bodt, M.S., Maryn, Y., Van de Heyning, P. and Hernandez-Diaz, M.E. (2007) Properties of the cepstral peak prominence and its usefulness in vocal quality measurements. Paper presented at MAVEBA '07, Florence.

Giovanni, A., Robert, D., Estublier, N., Teston, B., Zanaret, M. and Cannoni, M. (1996) Objective evaluation of dysphonia: Preliminary results of a device allowing simultaneous acoustic and aerodynamic measurements. *Folia Phoniatrica et Logopaedica* 48 (4), 175–185.

Hakkesteegt, M., Brocaar, M., Wieringa, M. and Feenstra, L. (2006) Influence of age and gender on the dysphonia severity index. A study of normative values. *Folia Phoniatrica et Logopaedica* 58 (4), 264–273.

Hakkesteegt, M.M., Brocaar, M.P., Wieringa, M.H. and Feenstra, L. (2008a) The relationship between perceptual evaluation and objective multiparametric evaluation of dysphonia severity. *Journal of Voice* 22 (2), 138–145.

Hakkesteegt, M., Wieringa, M., Brocaar, M., Mulder, P. and Feenstra, L. (2008b) The interobserver and test-retest variability of the dysphonia severity index. *Folia Phoniatrica et Logopaedica* 60 (2), 86–90.

Hakkesteegt, M.M., Brocaar, M.P. and Wieringa, M.H. (2010) The applicability of the Dysphonia Severity Index and the Voice Handicap Index in evaluating effects of voice therapy and phonosurgery. *Journal of Voice* 24 (2), 199–205.

Hirano, M. (1981) *Clinical Examination of Voice*. New York: Springer-Verlag.

Kempster, G.B., Gerratt, B.R., Verdolini Abbott, K., Barkmeier-Kraemer, J. and Hillman, R.E. (2009) Consensus auditory-perceptual evaluation of voice: Development of a standardized clinical protocol. *American Journal of Speech-Language Pathology* 18 (2), 124–132.

Kent, R.D. (1996) Hearing and believing: Some limits to the auditory-perceptual assessment of speech and voice disorders. *American Journal of Speech-Language Pathology* 5 (3), 7–23.

Kreiman, J. and Gerratt, B.R. (1998) Validity of rating scale measures of voice quality. *Journal of the Acoustical Society of America* 104, 1598–1608.

Ma, E.P.M. and Yiu, E.M.L. (2006) Multiparametric evaluation of dysphonic severity. *Journal of Voice* 20 (3), 380–390.

Maryn, Y., Dick, C., Vandenbruaene, C., Vauterin, T. and Jacobs, T. (2009a) Spectral, cepstral, and multivariate exploration of tracheoesophageal voice quality in continuous speech and sustained vowels. *Laryngoscope* 119 (12), 2384–2394.

Maryn, Y., Roy, N., De Bodt, M., Van Cauwenberge, P. and Corthals, P. (2009b) Acoustic measurement of overall voice quality: A meta-analysis. *Journal of the Acoustical Society of America* 126, 2619–2634.

Maryn, Y., Corthals, P., Van Cauwenberge, P., Roy, N. and De Bodt, M. (2010a) Toward improved ecological validity in the acoustic measurement of overall voice quality: Combining continuous speech and sustained vowels. *Journal of Voice* 24 (5), 540–555.

Maryn, Y., De Bodt, M. and Roy, N. (2010b) The Acoustic Voice Quality Index: Toward improved treatment outcomes assessment in voice disorders. *Journal of Communication Disorders* 43 (3), 161–174.

Piccirillo, J., Painter, C., Haiduk, A., Fuller, D. and Fredrickson, J. (1998) Assessment of two objective voice function indices. *Annals of Otology, Rhinology & Laryngology* 107 (5), 396–400.

Shrivastav, R. (2003) The use of an auditory model in predicting perceptual ratings of breathy voice quality. *Journal of Voice* 17 (4), 502–512.

Titze, I.R. (1994) *Principles of Voice Production.* Englewood Cliffs: Prentice-Hall.

Titze, I. (1995) *Summary Statement: Workshop on Acoustic Voice Analysis.* Denver: National Center for Voice and Speech.

Wolfe, V., Fitch, J. and Cornell, R. (1995) Acoustic prediction of severity in commonly occurring voice problems. *Journal of Speech and Hearing Research* 38 (2), 273–279.

Wolfe, V., Fitch, J. and Martin, D. (1997) Acoustic measures of dysphonic severity across and within voice types. *Folia Phoniatrica et Logopaedica* 49 (6), 292–299.

Wuyts, F.L., De Bodt, M.S., Bruckers, L. and Molenberghs, G. (1996) Research work of the Belgian Study Group on Voice Disorders 1996. Results. *Acta Oto-Rhino-Laryngologica Belgica* 50 (4), 331–341.

Wuyts, F.L., De Bodt, M.S., Molenberghs, G., Remacle, M., Heylen, L., Millet, B., *et al.* (2000) The dysphonia severity index: An objective measure of vocal quality based on a multiparameter approach. *Journal of Speech, Language, and Hearing Research* 43 (3), 796–809.

Yu, P., Ouaknine, M., Revis, J. and Giovanni, A. (2001) Objective voice analysis for dysphonic patients: A multiparametric protocol including acoustic and aerodynamic measurements. *Journal of Voice* 15 (4), 529–542.